# A GUIDE TO PSYCHOTHERAPY IN IRELAND

IRISH COUNCIL FOR PSYCHOTHERAPY

# A Guide to Psychotherapy in Ireland

## Third Revised Edition

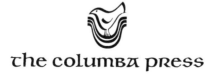

the columba press

This edition published in 2000

First edition published in 1997 by
**the columba press**

55A Spruce Avenue, Stillorgan Industrial Park,
Blackrock, Co Dublin


Cover by Bill Bolger
Origination by The Columba Press
Printed in Ireland by Colour Books Ltd., Dublin


ISBN 1 85607 291 6

# Contents

# EXECUTIVE COMMITTEE OF
# THE IRISH COUNCIL FOR PSYCHOTHERAPY

ELLEN O'MALLEY-ĐUNLOP
*Chair*

BARBARA FITZGERALD
*Honorary Secretary/Vice Chair*

TOM BREEN
*Honorary Treasurer*

MARGARET ĐALY
ICPA

ED MC HALE
FTAI

MARIA MC CARRON
CBT

ĐES MOORE
CBT

ANNE RICHARDSON
FTAI

BRION SWEENEY
ICPA

MARY-PAULA WALSH
IAHIP

## HONORARY MEMBERS
MICHAEL FITZGERALD
GER MURPHY
RUTH O'DONNELL

*Contact address:*

Irish Council for Psychotherapy
73 Quinn's Road,
Shankill,
Co Dublin.
Telephone: (01) 2722105
Fax: (01) 2722111
e-mail: amdps@indigo.ie

# ABBREVIATIONS FOR ORGANISATIONS

*CBT*       Cognitive Behavioural Therapy

*FTAI*      Family Therapy Association of Ireland

*IAHIP*     Irish Association of Humanistic and Integrative
            Psychotherapy

*ICPA*      Irish Constructivist Psychotherapy Association

*IFCAPP*    The Irish Forum for Child and Adolescent
            Psychoanalytic Psychotherapy

*IFPP*      The Irish Forum for Psychoanalytic Psychotherapy

*IGAS*      Irish Group Analytic Society

# Introduction

When a person is seeking the services of a psychotherapist, it is important to seek an experienced and well-trained psycho-therapist. The Irish Council for Psychotherapy is publishing this third edition of *A Guide to Psychotherapy in Ireland* to help the public choose the proper and appropriate help.

The Irish Council for Psychotherapy contains five sections, which represent different approaches within the psychotherapy field. They are:

Cognitive Behavioural Therapy
Constructivist Psychotherapy
Couple and Family Therapy
Humanistic and Integrative Psychotherapy
Psychoanalytic Psychotherapy

The *Guide* contains a brief description of each approach, which will identify some of the differences between the approaches, but we have found that psychotherapists of different orientations have more in common, in the manner in which they work, than they have differences. It is imperative that anyone seeking help should be assured that the person they are seeing is competent, committed and capable of the highest integrity in relation to the execution of their work. Each of the five sections has their own organisational structure, training standards, code of ethics and complaints and disciplinary procedures. The Register provides the names of professionals who have undergone an in depth training, and who are committed to upholding the high standards of professional conduct required by their section.

Psychotherapy is now just over one hundred years old. Apart from a long established psychoanalytic practice in Monkstown, Co Dublin, psychotherapy is relatively new in Ireland. Over the past twenty years, training programmes and psychotherapy services have become available here. Prior to this, those who wished to become psychotherapists had to go abroad for formal training, but thankfully many returned to work in Ireland and have become the pioneers in Ireland in psychotherapy training and practice. No longer have aspiring psychotherapists to go abroad as professional training in psychotherapy is now available in Ireland.

As with any new profession, it takes time to establish itself. Given the nature of the profession of psychotherapy in particular, the members are very aware of the need to be active in regulating both the trainings and the practice of psychotherapy, to safeguard public interest and to promote excellence in the profession overall. We continue to advise the Department of Health of the developments within our organisation and are active in lobbying for statutory registration for psychotherapists. In June 2000, the ICP had the honour of hosting the Ninth European Association for Psychotherapy Congress in UCD, Belfield, as our former Chairman Dr. Ed Mc Hale is the current President of the EAP. The Minister for Health, Mr. Mícheál Martin, officially opened the Congress and this augers well for future support for psychotherapy within the Department of Health.

As well as engaging in all the activities required by a professional organisation in Ireland, the ICP is a National Awarding Organisation of the European Association for Psychotherapy. The ICP has been involved in the development of the

European Certificate of Training in conjunction with the European Association for Psychotherapy, as well as the European Commission. The Commission promotes the recognition of common standards of training for psychotherapists throughout Europe, and will ensure their mobility across member states. While the European Commission does not have power to legally implement the certificate before it is adopted by member states, they have recommended it to the national co-ordinators of member states and welcome it as an initiative in establishing joint platforms which will facilitate the employment of migrants within the European Union.

This *Guide* will hopefully provide a useful source of reference for those who wish to know more about psychotherapy, and particularly for those who are considering using the services of appropriately trained and ethically responsible professionals, in addressing the issues in their personal lives and relationships.

ELLEN O'MALLEY-DUNLOP
Chair, ICP

# Ethical Guidelines of
# The European Association for Psychotherapy

*The present ethical guidelines were prepared by the standing advisory Ethics-Group of the EAP 1993-1995 and are validated in this version since 1995.*

## Preamble

In the practice of the therapeutic profession, all members of the EAP national associations, EAP member organisations, as well as EAP individual members, accept that the practice of psychotherapy requires responsibility in relation to their own persons, their psychotherapeutic tasks as well as towards clients who have entrusted themselves to a professional psychotherapist and with whom they have thus entered a special relationship. EAP member organisations are responsible for concerning themselves with ethical questions. This is applicable to trainers, members and trainees of these organisations.

The ethical guidelines of the national organisations serve:
- to protect the patients/clients from unethical applications of psychotherapy by all its psychotherapists and training members.
- to set standards for its members.
- as a foundation for the settling of complaints.

## 1. Applicability

The following ethical guidelines are binding on all member organisations of EAP as well as individual members. EAP member institutions are obliged to have their own ethical guidelines that are compatible with those of the EAP.

## 2. The Psychotherapeutic Profession

The psychotherapeutic profession is a separate scientific profession. It deals with the diagnosing and comprehensive, knowledgeable and planned treatment of psychosocially and/or psychosomatically derived behavioural disturbances or states of suffering by means of scientific and psychotherapeutic methods. The psychotherapeutic process is based upon the interaction between one or more patients/clients and one or more psychotherapists with the aim of facilitating changes and further development.

The psychotherapeutic profession is characterised by its commitment to the responsible accomplishment of the aforementioned aims.

Psychotherapists are required to use their expertise while taking into account the individual's dignity and esteem, for the patient's/client's best interest. Psychotherapists must declare their professional status and training, as appropriate.

## 3. Professional Competence and Development

Psychotherapists are required to practise their profession in a competent and ethical manner. They are required to pay attention to research and developments in the scientific field of psychotherapy. To achieve this, practitioners need to ensure their on-going professional development. Psychotherapists should limit their practice to those areas and treatment methods where it can be proven that they have gained sufficient and certified knowledge and experience.

## 4. Confidentiality

Psychotherapists, as well as all support staff, are bound by principles of confidentiality regarding all information that has become known to them during their psychotherapeutic involvement/practice. The same applies to supervision.

## 5. Frame Issues

At the beginning of the psychotherapeutic treatment, psychotherapists are required to make the patient/client aware of their rights with special emphasis on the following:

*The psychotherapeutic method employed (if appropriate and adequate to the process of the psychotherapeutic treatment) and the conditions (including the termination policy).

*Extent and probable duration of the psychotherapeutic treatment.

*Financial terms of the treatment (approximate fees, insurance claims, payment for missed sessions, etc.)

*Confidentiality.

*Complaints procedure.

The patient/client should be given the opportunity to decide whether they wish to enter psychotherapy and if so, with whom.

Psychotherapists are required to act responsibly, especially given the special nature of the psychotherapeutic relationship which is built on trust and a certain degree of dependency. Abuse and breach of trust is defined as psychotherapists' neglect of their professional responsibilities in relation to the patient/client in order to satisfy their own personal interests, be they sexual, emotional, social or financial. Any form of misuse is an offence against professional psychotherapeutic guidelines. The responsibility for this lies solely with the psychotherapist. Failure of responsibility in dealing with the trust and dependency relationship in psychotherapy is a serious error of treatment.

## 6. Factual/Objective and True Information

Information given to patients/clients must be factual/objective and true. Any blatant or misleading advertising is impermissible. Examples of this form of misleading and impermissible advertising could be: insupportable promises of healing or the quoting of many different types of psychotherapeutic methods (psychotherapeutic training begun without completion) which might give the impression of a more comprehensive or broader psychotherapeutic training than is the actual case.

### 7. Professional Relations with Colleagues

Psychotherapists, where necessary, are required to work interdisciplinarily with representatives of other professions for the well-being of the patient/client.

### 8. Ethical Guidelines for Training

The aforementioned ethical guidelines are also to be applied to the relationship between trainer and trainee, as appropriate.

### 9. Contribution to the Health Sector

As regards their social responsibility, psychotherapists are encouraged to make a contribution to the maintenance and creation of living conditions which will enhance, maintain and restore psychological health, and generally help further the maturity and development of people.

### 10. Psychotherapy Research

In the interest of the scientific-theoretical development of psychotherapy as well as psychotherapy outcome research, psychotherapists should participate in appropriate research projects. Psychotherapeutic research, as well as psychotherapy publications, are subject to the above ethical guidelines. The interests of the patients/clients are paramount.

### 11. Infringement of Ethical Guidelines

Each member organisation must have appropriate complaint and appeal procedures.

## 12. Duties of the National EAP Organisations

National organisations must require their practitioners to abide by codes of ethics that are compatible with EAP guidelines.

# PART I

# A National Register
# of Psychotherapists in Ireland

ALDERDICE, John
ANDREWS, Paul
ARNOLD, Mavis
ARTHURS, Mary
AYLWIN, Susan.
BAILEY, Jane
BAIRD, Jane
BANNON, John
BARRY, Kathleen
BARRY, Kay
BARRY, Myra
BAYLY, Kathrin
BEAUMONT, Margaret
BEIRNE, Rosarii
BENNETT, Eamon
BENSON, Jarlath
BERGIN, Alexander.
BERMINGHAM, Anne
    Marie
BERMINGHAM, Paula
BOGGINS, Tom
BOLAND, Emille
BONFIELD, Dymphna
BOROSON, Martin
BOURKE, Carmel
BOYLE, Martin
BOYNE, Edward
BREEN, Noreen
BREEN, Tom
BREHONY, Rita

BRENT, Rebecca
BRIGHT, Jill
BROPHY, John
BROPHY, Margaret T.M.
BROSNAN, Joan
BROWNE, Essie
BROWNE, Larry
BUCKLEY, Marguerite
BUCKLEY, Marion
BUCKLEY, Triona
BURBRIDGE, Paul
BURKE, Phil
BURNS, Maura
BURSTALL, Taru
BUTCHER, Gerard
BUTLER, Goretti
BUTLER, Maggie
BUTLER, Pauline
BYRNE, Carmel
BYRNE, Gerard
BYRNE, Kathleen
BYRNE, Mary
BYRNE, Nollaig
BYRNE, Padraic
BYRNE, Patrick
BYRNE, Tim
BYRNE, Ruth
CADWELL, Nuala
CAHILL, Michelle
CALLANAN, Fiodhna

CALLANAN, William
CAMPBELL, Carmel
CANAVAN, Catherine
CANAVAN, Mary
CARBERRY, Brian
CARPENTER, Anne
CARR, Alan
CARROLL, Anna
CARROLL, Patricia
CARTON, Simone
CASEY, Grainne.
CASSERLY, Felicity
CHILDERS, Nessa
CHOISEUL, Anne
CLAFFEY, Elaine
CLANCY, Mary
CLARKE, Margaret
CLARKE, Michelle
COGHLAN, Helena
COLEMAN, Padraig
COLGAN, Patrick J.
COLLEARY, Maura
COLLINS, Barbara
COLLINS, Deirdre
COLLINS, Geraldine
COLLINS, Ines
COLLINS, Mary
COLLINS-SMYTH,
     Margaret
COMERFORD, Anna
CONAGHAN, Mary
CONNEELY, Caitlin
CONNOLLY, Brendan
CONNOLLY, Brendan M.
CONNOLLY, Margaret
CONROY, Kay
COSTELLO, Margaret
COTTER, Donald
COUGHLAN, Helena

COX, Ann
COX, Olga
COYLE, Brigid
CROWLEY, Betty
CULLEN, Mary
CUNNINGHAM, Kathy
CUNNINGHAM, Nora
CURTIN, Gerardine
DALY, Margaret
DALY, Martin
DALY, Martin J.
DARBY, Mary
DAVEY, Damien
DE BURCA, Bairbre
DE JONGH, Corry.
DE LACY, Mara.
DEENY, Margaret
DEERY, Pat
DELAHUNTY, Alan
DELMONTE, Michael M.
DENENY, Mary
DENNEHY, Noreen
DEVLIN, Fiona
DEVLIN, Teresa
DIBBLE, Annie
DILLON, Marie
DOCKERY, Bernadette
DOHERTY, Myra
DONNELLY, Pat.
DONOGHUE, Mary
DONOHOE, Eugene
DONOHOE, Mary
DOODY, Brendan
DOOLEY, Deirdre
DORR, Frank
DOWD, Teresa
DOWLING, Brenda
DOWNEY, Betty
DOYLE, Grainne

DOYLE, Mary
DOYLE, Rosaleen
DOYLE, Sherry
DRISCOLL, Angela
DRISCOLL, Zelie
DU LAING, Annemie
DUFFY, Kathleen
DUFFY, Martin
DUFFY, Mary
DUGGAN, Colman.
DUGGAN, Noel.
DULLAGHAN, Elizabeth
  (Lillie).
DUNCAN, Audrey
DUNLEA, Marian
DUNNE, Ann Maria
DUNNE, Patricia
DWYER, Frankie-Ann
DYKES, Teresa
EGAN, Angela
EGAN, Barbara
ELLIS, Mary
FADDEN, Rosaleen
FAHY, Bernadette
FAHY, Michael
FAY, Joe
FERRITER, Kay
FINGLETON, May
FINLAYSON, Douglas
FINNEGAN, Leo
FITZGERALD, Ann
FITZGERALD, Barbara
FITZGERALD, Michael
FITZMAURICE, John
FLEMING, Pearl
FLYNN, Deirdre
FLYNN, Madeleine
FLYNN, Stephen
FOGARTY, Geraldine

FOLEY, Dermot
FOLEY, Miriam
FOLEY, Robert
FORBES, Jean
FORDE, Angela
FORREST, Mary
FOX, Michael
FOY, Emma
FRASER, Teresa
FRAWLEY, Angela
FRAWLEY, Michael
FRENCH, Gerry
FULTON, Linda
GAFFNEY, Delia
GALLIGAN, Patricia
GANLEY, Brian
GARLAND, Clive
GILL, Anne
GILL, Margaret
GILLILAND, Kay
GILMARTIN, Helen
GLEESON, Betty
GORDON, Evelyn
GRIEVE, Karin
GRIMLEY, Carmel
GRINDLEY, Geraldine
GROSSMAN FREYNE, Gail
GROVER, Mary
GUNNE, David
GUNNE, Dorothy
HAGAN, Patricia
HAMILL, Carmel
HARGIN, Mary Rose
HARNEY, Vivian
HARRINGTON, Eileen
HAUGHEY, Monica
HAYES, Fran
HEALY, Anette
HEALY, Daniel

REGISTER

HEALY, Donal
HEDIGAN, Helen
HEFFERNAN, Michael
HEGARTY, Donal
HEGARTY, Owen
HEGARTY, Tony
HENNIGAN, Cecily
HERLIHY, Mary P.
HESKIN, Christina
HILL, Rosemary
HIRST, Iain
HOGAN-FLEMING, Bernie
HOLLAND, Joanna
HOLLAND, Mary
HOMAN, Anne Marie
HONNAY, Emiel
HORNER, Carol
HORNER, Philomena
HOULIHAN, Tom
HOWARD, Leslie
HOWLETT, Brian
HUGHES, Maria
HUMPHREYS, Vincent
HUNTER, Alison I.
IRWIN, Edith
JACKSON, Ann
JACKSON, Caitriona
JEBB, Winston
JEFFRIES, Mary
JENNINGS, Norman
JONES, Coleen
JONES, Helen
JOYCE, Nora
JUDGE, Jimmy
JUTHAN, Kay
KAVANAGH, Ann
KAY, Sarah
KEANE, Verena
KEARNEY, Philip

KEARNEY, Ruth
KEELAN, Annette
KEENAN, Marie
KEHOE, Helen
KEIGHER, Marian
KELLEHER, Kathleen
KELLIHER, Anne
KELLY, Valerie
KELTNER-HOLLAND,
    Joanna
KENNEDY, Jo
KENNY, Vincent
KIERNAN, Donal
KILCOYNE, Phyllis
KILGALLEN, Aideen
KILLORAN-GANNON,
    Sheila
KILMARTIN, Annie
KING, Margaret
KIRK, Geraldine
KLOPP, Marianne
KOHNSTAMM, Barbara
LALOR, Mary
LANIGAN, Nora
LAWLOR, Mary Brigid
LAWLOR, Paula
LEE, Mary
LESLIE, Frank
LEWIS, Maeve
LIDDY, Rosemary
LINDEN, Mairead
LINDSAY, John
LINDSAY, Susan
LINNANE, Paul
LOGAN, Paddy
LONERGAN, Mary-Anna
LOUGHLIN, Paula
LUCEY, Joe
LYNCH, Barbara

LYNCH, Catherine
LYNCH, Eileen
LYONS, Sheila
MAC GUINNESS, Irene
MAC NEILL, Sile
MACNAMARA, Vincent
MADDEN, Joan
MADDEN, Louise
MAGEE, David
MAGENIS, Maire
MAGUIRE, Maura
MAGUIRE, Una
MAHER, Ann
MAHER, Bonnie
MAHER, Pascal
MAIR, Bridget Marie
MANDOS, Koos
MANGAN, Mary
MANNION WALSHE,
    Deirdre
MARTIN, Maeve
MARTIN, Raymond
MASTERSON, Ingrid
MATHEWS, Peter
MAWN, Kate
MC ADAM, Frank
MC ALEER, Jennifer
MC CABE, Nancy
MC CARRICK, Tom
MC CARTHY, Aine
MC CARTHY, Angela
MC CARTHY, Anne
MC CARTHY, Dan
MC CARTHY, Eunice
MC CARTHY, Imelda
MC CARTHY, Patricia
MC CARTHY, Rita
MC CARTHY, Ros
MC CASHIN, Dolores

MC CLOAT, Catherine
MC CONALOGUE,
    Margaret
MC CORMACK, Marijke
MC COURT, Ann
MC COURT, Marie
MC CULLY, Maria
MC DONNELL, Patricia
MC FADDEN, Hugh
MC GEE, Annette
MC GEE, Breda
MC GEE, David
MC GLYNN, James
MC GLYNN, Peter
MC GOLDRICK, Mary
MC GRATH, Terri
MC GROARY-MEEHAN,
    Maureen
MC GUINNESS, Sharon
MC HALE, Edmund
MC HUGH, Charles
MC KEE, Catherine Anne
MC KEE, Maud
MC KEON, Lindsay
MC LEAVEY, Bernadette
MC LOONE, Anne
MC LOUGHLIN, Maire
MC LOUGHLIN, Sarah
MC MANUS, Libby
MC MORROW, Mary
MC QUAID, Margaret
MEAGHER, Kathleen A.
MEEK, Pauline
MELVIN PERREM, Joan
MERNAGH, Elizabeth
MICHAEL, Joan
MOHALLY, Derry
MOLEY, Patrick
MONAGHAN, Ann

MONGEY, Sile
MOONEY, Jennifer
MOONEY MC GLOIN,
    Catherine
MOORE, Des
MOORE, Lucy
MORRISON, Anne
MORRISSEY, Germaine
MOUNTAIN, Jane
MOYLAN, Bernadette
MULHERE, Jacinta
MULHOLLAND, Marie
    Therese
MULLER, Elisabeth
MULLIGAN, Kathleen
MURNANE, Eilis
MURPHY, Ann C.
MURPHY, Brendan
MURPHY, David
MURPHY, Ger
MURPHY, John
MURPHY, Mary
MURPHY, Mary
MURPHY, Mary
MURPHY, Patricia
MURPHY, Ruth
MURPHY, Zoe
MURRAY, Claire
MURRAY, Denis
MURRAY, Janet
MURRAY, Marie
MURRAY, Mary
MYERS, Gerard
NANNERY, Teresa
NAUGHTON, Anne Marie
NEARY, Nora
NEVIN, Peter
NEWMAN, Josephine
NÍ GHALLCHOBHAIR,

Maighréad
NÍ NUALLÁIN, Máirín
NÍ UALLACHÁIN, Méabh
NIC DHOMHNAILL,
    Caoimhe
NOLAN, Bernadette
NOLAN, Declan
NOLAN, Inger
NOLAN, Patrick
NORMAND, Tessa
NOWLAN, Kate
O'BRIEN, Anne
O'BRIEN, David
O'BRIEN, Gay
O'BRIEN, Jim
O'BRIEN, Margaret
O'BRIEN, Tom
O'BRIEN, Valerie
O'BYRNE, Celine
O'CONNELL, Patricia
O'CONNOR, Aine
O'CONNOR, Colm J.
O'CONNOR, Elizabeth
O'CONNOR, Karen E.
O'CONNOR, Marika
O'CONNOR, Mary Rose
O'DALAIGH, Liam
O'DEA, Catherine
O'DEA, Eileen
O'DOHERTY, Colm
O'DONNELL, Godfrey
O'DONNELL, Ruth
O'DONOGHUE, Eilis
O'DONOGHUE, Jim
O'DONOGHUE, Paul
O'DONOVAN, Joan
O'DONOVAN, Mairin
O'DONOVAN, Margot
O'DOWD, Maura

O'DUFFY, Ann
O'DWYER, Mary
O'FARRELL, Magda
O'FLAHERTY, Anne
O'GRADY, Bernadette
O'GRADY, Ethna
O'GRADY, Paul
O'HALLORAN, Mary
O'HALLORAN, Michael
O'HANLON, Judy
O'HARA, Carmel
O'HORA, Claire
O'HORA, Nollaig
O'LEARY, Eleanor
O'LOCHLIN, Theresa
O'MAHONY, Berenice
O' MAHONY, Catherine
O'MAHONY, Eileen
O'MAHONY, Hank
O'MAHONY, Judy
O'MAHONY, Kathleen
O'MALLEY, Grace
O'MALLEY-DUNLOP, Ellen
O'NEILL, Ann
O'NEILL, Breege
O'NEILL, Deborah
O'NEILL, Elizabeth
O'NEILL, Julia
O'NEILL, Mary
O'NEILL, Nora
O'REILLY, Aine
O'REILLY, Joseph
O'REILLY, Maureen
O'ROURKE, Darina
O'SCOLLAIN, Eibhlin
O'SHAUGHNESSY, Marie
O'SHEA, Deirdre
O'SULLIVAN, Ann
O'SULLIVAN, Bernadette

O'SULLIVAN, Creina
O'SULLIVAN, Marych
O'SULLIVAN, Rita
O'TOOLE, Muriel
OWENS, Conor
PARKS, Ann
PEAKIN, Anne
PERREM, Breda
PHALAN, Sally
PORTER, Sheila
PRENDERVILLE, Mary
PRICE, Noeleen
PRYLE, Fiona M.
PURCELL, Rosanna
PYLE, Mary
RABBETT, Marie
REIDY, Margaret
REYNOLDS, Mary
RICHARDSON, Anne
RICHARDSON, Colette
RIGNEY, Jeanette
RINTOUL, Irene
RIORDAN, Gillian
ROCHE, Anne
ROCHE, Declan
ROCHE, Freda
ROCHE, Sile
ROE, Liam
ROTHERY, Nuala
RUSSELL, Maura
RUTH, Ann
RYAN, Ann
RYAN, Anne
RYAN, Catherine
RYAN, David
RYAN, Derval
RYAN, Mairead
RYAN, Teresa
RYAN, Toni

REGISTER

SAHAFI, Janet E.
SAMPSON, Annie
SCIASCIA, Dolores
SCULLY, Mary
SCULLY, Patricia
SCULLY, Rosaleen
SELL, Patrick
SHEEHAN, Bartley
SHEEHAN, Helen
SHEEHAN, Jim
SHEEHAN, Mary
SHEEHAN, Thomas
SHEILL, Mary
SHERIDAN, Anne
SHIELDS, Vivienne
SHORTEN, Karen
SKAR, Patricia
SKELTON, Ross
SMITH, Mary
SMITH, Ray
SMITH, Susan
SMYTH, Geraldine
SOMERS, Olive
SPARROW, Bobbie
STAUNTON, Pauline
STEFANAZZI, Mary
STONE, William
SWAIN, Ronny
SWEENEY, Brion
SWEENEY, Delma
SWEENEY, Irene
SWEENEY, Patrick
TANSEY, Louise

TIERNEY, Aileen
TIERNEY, Margaret
TIGHE, Jacinta
TONE, Yvonne
TROOP, Deborah
TYRRELL, Patricia
UNDERWOOD-QUINN,
     Nicola
VAN DOORSLAER, Mia
VAN HOUT, Els
WADE, Richard
WALL MURPHY, Maura
WALLACE, Carmel
WALLACE, George
WALSH, Angela
WALSH, Mary-Paula
WALSHE, Siobhan
WALSHE, Tony
WARD, Mary B.
WARD, Shirley
WARDEN, Norman
WATSON, Patricia
WEATHERILL, Rob
WHITE, Joan
WIECZOREK-DEERING,
     Dorit
WILLIAMS, Jane
WILSDON, Sheelagh
WOODS, Jean
WRIXON GOGGIN, Pauline
WYLIE-WARREN, Frances
YOUNG, Anne
YOUNG, Sheilagh

# PART II

# Approaches to Psychotherapy

## Cognitive-Behavioural Psychotherapy (CBT)

The philosophical underpinning of this approach is that a person learns to act and think in certain ways as a result of their experiences and their perceptions of those experiences. This learning is a life-long process. Usually what we learn is adaptive and functional – we learn to become active participants in our lives, our society and our culture. However, occasionally we learn ways of thinking, feeling or behaving which hinder us in our development and prevent us from achieving our potential. Sometimes a single event such as being bitten by a dog, or a car crash, will have major repercussions; or, more often, experiences which go over a longer period of time, e.g. being bullied or being unemployed can affect us emotionally in the long term. Such negative experiences and responses to them can lead us to develop low self-esteem, unhappiness, bitterness, anxiety, passivity, aggression, perfectionism and so on. These, in turn, colour the way we perceive new experiences and at worst, if unchecked, can lead to such disorders as clinical depression, eating disorders, obsessive-compulsive disorder and panic disorder.

Clients present with a variety of different problems from a wide span of human experiences. Clients with a learning disability are helped to play a full part in society by extra teaching for the individual through a process of behaviour analysis. Each individual has the same rights and needs as everyone else in society. These clients' needs can be compounded due to physical disabilities, behavioural problems or communication deficits. Methods need to be used consistently within a particular context, by all of those involved, including the carer of the client who may have their own needs on a practical and emotional level. This approach examines people's behaviours in their living environment. It identifies the function challenging behaviour, services the individual, the source of the behaviour and its maintenance.

Clients experiencing stress and anxiety with marked avoidance behaviour (behaviour which postpones an anxiety evoking event and can lead to handicaps in every day life) can change their way of acting, e.g. become more outgoing and combat their fears with the help of individualised tailored Behaviour Therapy programmes.

They may have to confront repeatedly what they fear, e.g., contamination fear where the sufferer avoids certain perceived contaminated objects, progressing from the least feared object to the most feared. Personal accountability is the key to the client overcoming their problem. Motivation to complete home-work assignments and record progress between sessions, facilitates the carry-over into their daily lives of the skills and insights achieved by the client during therapy. This intervention and the willingness to explore new coping strategies are the ingredients for success.

Whereas in the past, Behaviour Therapy dealt only with what was observable, i.e. actions and behaviours, assuming rightly that once these were changed, thoughts and feelings would change to match the new behaviours. The cognitive therapists postulated that people can achieve change by working directly on their own patterns of thinking. Just as we may have, through our life experiences, learnt distorted patterns of thought (patterns which hinder rather than help), so can we learn new, helpful and functional thought patterns. The way we think impacts on every aspect of our lives, from hopefulness regarding the future, to personal relationships, to how we see ourselves and everything in between.

Cognitive and behavioural interventions overlap in their shared purpose of loosening the hold a particular negative belief has on the client and engaging him in a re-evaluation of his perceptions and assumptions.

The progress of the therapy is interactive. Its axis is in a relationship between the client and the therapist. The therapist uses a systematic framework that recognises the client as an individual and his/her need to be a participant in the solution to their own problems. People who experience interpersonal difficulties can benefit from group work using the key characteristics of the cognitive behavioural approach:

* assessment/analysis of the problem
* creating a therapeutic alliance
* agreed therapy goals and targets
* regular measurement and evaluation of progress towards targets.

Assessment is individual for each client. It involves detailed questioning and the use of psychological questionnaires to enable the client and therapist to define accurately the problem and set the goals of treatment. Cognitive-behavioural psychotherapy concentrates on the present – how we are now. It is practical and pragmatic, a collaborative effort by the therapist and client working together, rather like an investigative team; and is based on sound empirical findings. The aim of therapy is to provide the client with knowledge and techniques which he/she can use now and in the future, in effect, making the therapist redundant. Therapy is time limited and can be individual, family or group. Group treatment includes:

Assertiveness, Stress Management, Anger Management and Social Skills Training. Each client is given a detailed account of treatment options and their consent is sought before embarking on therapy. Registered practitioners adhere to a code of ethics, and are committed to research and the development of theory within this sphere.

Overall, practitioners use the developing pool of knowledge in this field to resolve problems of living for any person, irrespective of intelligence or insight.

*Contact address:*   Jacinta Mulhere, CBT,
St Vincent's Centre,
Navan Road,
Dublin 7.
Tel: (01) 8383234 Ext. 120

### *List of Practitioners*

*For addresses and telephone numbers, please refer to the Directory section.*

BARRY, Kathleen
BENNETT, Eamonn
BURBRIDGE, Paul
BURKE, Phil
DEVLIN, Teresa
DOHERTY, Myra
FITZMAURICE, John
HARNEY, Vivian
MATHEWS, Peter
MC ADAM, Frank
MC FADDEN, Hugh.

MC GLYNN, Jim
MC GOLDRICK, Mary
MC GROARY-MEEHAN, Maureen
MC GUINNESS, Sharon
MOONEY MC GLOIN, Catherine
MOORE, Des
MULHERE, Jacinta
RYAN, Mairead
TONE, Yvonne

# Family Therapy (FTAI)

*What is special about Family Therapy?*

Family Therapy is the most popularly recognised descriptive title for a body of practice and theory which continues to evolve and to grow at an extraordinary rate. Originally, the approach was distinguished by the practice of including entire families in the therapy process rather than an individual client. This practice continues, but is not a necessary aspect of the approach. The principle which informed Family Therapy from the time of its inception in the 1950s has been to transcend simple cause and effect explanations which located deficits within the individual, and to include those aspects of the client's context in the therapy process which will enable them to manage, resolve or better understand their difficulty. It is this ecological view which attends to the interconnectedness of people, of beliefs and of all things, which characterises Family Therapy rather than the number of people sitting in the therapy room.

*How do Family Therapists view problems and reality?*

Many Family Therapists seek to engage the clients in a collaborative exploration of their presenting dilemma, focusing on the beliefs, and the interactions which maintain the difficulty or which prevent its resolution. By better understanding the interconnectedness of the biological, the social and the psychological dimensions of the problem, choices are introduced, conflicts are transcended and new patterns of understanding are generated.

A significant part of each one's experience is the beliefs, the language, the stories and values which constitute our life experience. We are not only born into a material and physical reality, but also into a multilayered complex weave of beliefs and behaviours, which for most of us are, initially at least, of a family nature. This strongly influences our developing 'reality'. We are born into the world totally dependent on one or more caring adults, and if the constitutional and contextual aspects of our lives are supportive enough, we learn to operate more independently and to exercise choice in our lives more effectively. This requires an appreciation of the interdependence of our lives, of the world in which we live, and the limits and possibilities which it contains. We constantly explore the limits and possibilities of relying on previous learning and exploring new ways and new beliefs. We may be strongly influenced to find ways of being which contrast with some of our significant life experiences, or we may repeat our experiences, often with the assumption that this is how the world is, and how everyone should be.

When two or more people live in close proximity, we can expect that differences, and inevitably conflicts, will ensue. This is part of the rich weave of our lives which continue to challenge us and to teach us.

Sometimes, our adult lives may be thrown into inner turmoil, we may experience self-doubts, destructive feelings or immobilising depression or anxiety. These disturbing experiences may be triggered by what would be relatively small or manageable difficulties for others, and even for ourselves in somewhat different circumstances. Such problems are frequently related to early life and usually early family aspects of our lives. Our difficulty trusting others, exercising choice or living with an adequate level of autonomy may be related to not having had sufficiently secure, loving or affirming experiences in our early family relationships. More recent traumas, abuse, oppression or unresolved conflict may also contribute to distressing inner feelings, which can be successfully resolved in Family Therapy.

### What do Family Therapists do?

Family Therapists universally employ the most inclusive frame to help clients make sense of their doubts or confusions.

Some Family Therapists put most emphasis on exploring the beliefs, some the language and stories and some the repeating behaviour patterns. They may also elect to examine the attempted solutions or to focus attention on experiences which work well for the client, their successful solutions.

### How many attend Family Therapy together?

The extent to which Family Therapists will emphasise including others in the process also varies. With relationship problems, we usually prefer to include the main participants. It is not uncommon for parents to successfully attend a series of consultations regarding one of their children, without the child being present. Extended family members may be invited or partners or others who are significantly involved in the client's life and difficulty. It is also common for individuals to attend alone, when the focus will include the significant relationships of their lives as the context of their emotional and psychological realities. Agreeing who will attend is usually an integral part of the exploratory process.

Some Family Therapists may also apply their systemic perspective to organisations such as schools, voluntary agencies, businesses and especially to family businesses. Consultation can help organisations to resolve intra organisations relationship problems and to address and to improve procedures and practices which influence their relationship with their consumers. The systemic consultant's focus will, again, include the context of the problem and can result in appreciating and

APPROACHES

fine tuning the ways in which the organisation responds to internal change and the range of changing external needs. The organisation, as the individual, can benefit by developing capacities of self-direction and responsivity.

*Contact address:*  The Secretary, FTAI,
                    73, Quinn's Road,
                    Shankill,
                    Co Dublin.
                    Tel: (01) 2722105

### *List of Practitioners*

*For addresses and telephone numbers, please refer to the Directory section.*

| | |
|---|---|
| BANNON, John | DE LACY, Mara |
| BAYLY, Kathrin | DELAHUNTY, Alan |
| BOURKE, Carmel | DENNEHY, Noreen |
| BROPHY, John | DOCKERY, Bernadette |
| BROWNE, Essie | DOOLEY, Deirdre |
| BUCKLEY, Marguerite | DOWNEY, Betty |
| BUTLER, Goretti | DRISCOLL, Zelie |
| BYRNE, Nollaig | DUFFY, Mary |
| BYRNE, Patrick | DUGGAN, Colman |
| CADWELL, Nuala | FADDEN, Rosaleen |
| CALLANAN, William | FAY, Joe |
| CARBERRY, Brian | FINGLETON, May |
| CARR, Alan | FITZGERALD, Barbara |
| CARROLL, Patricia | FORREST, Mary |
| CARTON, Simone | FRASER, Teresa |
| CLARKE, Michele | FRYER, Anthony |
| COLLINS, Geraldine | FULTON, Linda |
| COLLINS, Ines | GAFFNEY, Delia |
| CONNEELY, Caitlin | GALLIGAN, Claire |
| CONNOLLY, Brendan | GALLIGAN, Patricia |
| COSTELLO, Margaret T. | GILLILAND, Kay P. |
| DALY, Martin | GLEESON, Betty |
| DE JONGH, Corry | GORDON, Evelyn |

GROSSMAN FREYNE, Gail
GUNNE, Dorothy
HAYES, Fran
HEGARTY, Donal
HENNIGAN, Cecily
HIRST, Iain J.
HOLLAND, Mary
HORNER, Philomena
HOULIHAN, Tom
HOWARD, Leslie
JEBB, Winston.
JUTHAN, Kay.
KEANE, Verena
KEARNEY, Philip
KEENAN, Marie
KEIGHER, Marian
KELLEHER, Kathleen
KELLY, Valerie
KENNEDY, Jo
KILCOYNE, Phyllis
KIRK, Geraldine
KOHNSTAMM, Barbara
LALOR, Mary
LEE, Mary
LESLIE, Frank
LINNANE, Paul
LYONS, Sheila
MAC GUINNESS, Irene
MADDEN, Joan
MAGENIS, Maire
MAGUIRE, Maura
MAHER, Pascal
MANDOS, Koos
MC ALEER, Jennifer
MC CARTHY, Imelda
MC CARTHY, Ros
MC CONALOGUE, Margaret
MC GEE, Breda
MC HALE, Edmund

MC KEE, Anne
MC LOUGHLIN, Maire
MC LOUGHLIN, Sarah
MC MANUS, Libby
MC MORROW, Mary
MEEK, Pauline
MOLEY, Patrick
MONAGHAN, Ann
MONAGHAN, Theresa
MOORE, Lucy M.
MORRISON, Anne
MULHOLLAND, Marie-
  Therese
MURNANE, Eilis
MURPHY, Mary
MURPHY, Ruth
MURPHY, Trish
MURRAY, Denis
MURRAY, Marie
NOLAN, Inger
O'BRIEN, Gay
O'BRIEN, Jim
O'BRIEN, Margaret
O'BRIEN, Tom
O'BRIEN, Valerie
O'CONNOR, Colm
O'DALAIGH, Liam
O'DEA, Eileen
O'DONNELL, Ruth
O'DONOVAN, Mairin
O'GRADY, Ethna
O'HARA, Carmel
O'MAHONY, Eileen
O'MALLEY-DUNLOP, Ellen
O'NEILL, Breege
O'NEILL, Elizabeth
O'SCOLLAIN, Eibhlin
O'SHAUGHNESSY, Marie
O'SHEA, Deirdre

O'SULLIVAN, Bernadette
O'SULLIVAN, Creina
PORTER, Sheila
PRICE, Noeleen M.
PRYLE, Fiona M.
RICHARDSON, Anne
RICHARDSON, Colette
ROCHE, Declan
ROCHE, Freda
ROCHE, Sile
ROE, Liam
SCIASCIA, Dolores
SCULLY, Mary
SCULLY, Patricia
SHEEHAN, Jim

SHEEHAN, Tom
SHERIDAN, Anne
SHIELDS, Vivienne
SMITH, Susan
SWEENEY, Patrick
TROOP, Deborah
TYRRELL, Patricia M.
UNDERWOOD-QUINN,
 Nicola
WALL MURPHY, Maura
WALSH, Angela
WHITE, Joan
WHYTE, Monica
WILLIAMS, Jane
YOUNG, Sheilagh M.

APPROACHES

# Humanistic and Integrative Psychotherapy (IAHIP)

Therapists from a Humanistic and Integrative perspective invite people to develop their awareness as to what prevents them from unfolding their own true nature in the inner and outer expressions of their life.

*Historical Context*

The Humanistic Psychology movement developed in the 1960s in America out of a need to counter-balance the strong idealogical schools of scientific positivistic behaviourism and Freudian psychoanalysis. Both these ideological approaches to the person excluded some of the most important questions that make the human being human; for example, choice, values, love, creativity, self-awareness and human potential.

Yalom[1] makes an interesting observation as to the two strands underpinning the study of the nature of the person at that time, in both the European and American context. He says,

> '...it is interesting to note that the field of Humanistic Psychology developed alongside the 1960s counter culture in America with its attendant social phenomena such as the free speech movement, the flower children, the drug culture, the human potentialists and the sexual revolution', whereas '... the underpinnings of the European tradition of existentialist enquiry into the nature of the person was different. The existentialist position focused instead on human limitations and the tragic dimensions of existence'.[1]

This was partly shaped out of the society and culture at that time which had had a relatively recent history of war and geographic and ethnic confinement.

APPROACHES

In contrast, the human potential movement was 'bathed in a zeitgeist of expansiveness, optimism, limitless horizons and pragmatism'.[1] The European existentialist tradition focused on limits, on facing and taking into oneself the anxiety of uncertainty and non-being, whereas the Human Potential movement spoke less of limits and contingency than of development of potential, less of acceptance than of awareness, less of anxiety than of peak experiences and oceanic oneness, less of life meaning than of self-realization, less of apartness and basic isolation than of I-Thou encounter.

These two strands of thought emphasise the fact that any attempt to describe the person merely as a part needs to include the whole, and that the human story and nature of the person is always articulated within the wider social and cultural context of which that person is a part.

*The Nature of Humanistic and Integrative Psychotherapy*

Within the Humanistic and Integrative approach, some commonly held assumptions about the human person are as follows:

- *the individual is seen as a whole person living out their present level of integration through their body, feelings, mind, psyche and spirit.*

- *a person has responsibility for his/her life and for the choices they make.* People are responsible not only for their actions but for their failures to act. A metaphorical way to describe this is to reflect on a person inhabiting themselves, not so much as a concrete structure embedded in stone, but more like a web spun by the shaping of their inner and outer life, which can be spun again in any number of ways.

- *Humanistic and Integrative psychotherapy is based on a phenomenological view of reality.* Its emphasis is on experience. Therapists within this perspective frequently engage active techniques to encourage the deepening of the therapeutic process. There is a movement away from the goal of understanding events towards the active exploration of experience.

- *The nature of the person is seen as dynamic.* The person is seen as unfolding in different stages. There is always a thrust towards wholeness and life, but sometimes along the way, at any one stage, an overwhelming failure or frustration can be experienced as anxiety, depression or even a vague sense of an unlived life. These experiences can impede the emergence of later stages or result in an uneven integration as the person develops. Within each stage, different structures of relating to life emerge. Later structures transcend but include earlier ones, so that a question a person poses as they begin therapy, may be rooted in or have an echo in their earlier shaping, but will always include a harmonious note of future possibilities.

We stretch to where we need to stretch, and what a humanistic and integrative therapist does is to be continually present to the unfolding nature and quest of the person within the therapeutic setting.

### The Nature of the Therapeutic Process

Humanistic and Integrative therapies have many broad and creative approaches to working with clients. The therapeutic relationship is seen as a meaningful contract between equals, and the aims of therapy may be as diverse as encouraging the self-healing capacities of the client, to an exploration of a client's concrete individual experience of anxiety and distress rooted in earlier relationships, to an encouragement of insight into repeating patterns of behaviour which might be preventing clients from leading fulfilling and satisfying lives.

APPROACHES

The attitude and presence of the therapist is important. Yalom[2] speaks about the therapist entering into the client's experiential world and listening to the phenomena of that world without the pre-suppositions that distort understanding. Carl Rogers[3] focused on the importance of deep, attentive listening on the part of the therapist in promoting change.

*Integrative Aspects*

Practitioners in this field come from a range of perspectives on what it means to be a person. Some emphasise the body aspects, other the experiential feeling life and awareness of the person presenting, and others the wider contexts of meaning of which that person is a part.

The integrative approach emphasises the validity of a variety of approaches to the individual, and whilst remaining respectful to each approach, draws from many sources in the belief that no one approach has the whole truth.

Therapists are always guided by the respect and acceptance of the client as a whole person who has the potential to change, heal and grow.

*Irish Association of Humanistic and Integrative Psychotherapy*

The Irish Association of Humanistic and Integrative Psychotherapy was formed in 1992 as an association to represent Humanistic and Integrative psychotherapists in Ireland. In 1994, the I.A.H.I.P. became a company, limited by guarantee, and is one of the five psychotherapy sections of the Irish Council for Psychotherapy.

The aims of the I.A.H.I.P. are to set and maintain standards of training and practice, and to accredit suitably qualified practitioners of psychotherapy. Members adhere to a code of ethics and practice which includes a complaints procedure.

APPROACHES

*Contact address:*  The Secretary, IAHIP,
44, Northumberland Avenue,
Dun Laoghaire,
Co Dublin.
Tel: (01) 2841665

*Notes*

1. Yalom, Irwin D., *Existential Psychotherapy*, (Basic Books Inc., New York 1980).

2. *op. cit.* page 17.

3. Rogers, C., *On becoming a Person*, (Constable 1961).
— *Client-Centred Therapy*, (Constable 1965).
Further descriptions of Carl Rogers' work is contained in: Kirschenbaum, H. and Henderson, V. (eds), *The Carl Rogers Reader*, (Constable 1990).

*Further Reading:*

Rowan, J., *The Reality Game*, (Routledge & Keegan Paul, London 1983).
— *Subpersonalities*, (Routledge, London, 1990).
— *Ordinary Ecstasy*, (2nd Edition, 1988).
— *Humanistic Psychology in Action*, (Routledge, London).
— *The Transpersonal Psychotherapy and Counselling*, (Routledge, London, 1993).
Perls, F, Hefferline, R & Goodman, P., *Gestalt Therapy*, (Souvenir Press 1974).
Boadella, D., *Biosynthesis* (Routlege & Keegan Paul, 1987).
Lowen, A., *The Language of the Body*, (First Earlier Books, 1971).
Keleman, Stanley., *Emotional Anatomy* (Berkley, CA: Center Press, 1985).
Assagioli, R., *Psychosynthesis: A Manual of Principles and Techniques*, (Turnstone Books, 1980).
Wilber, K., *Eye to Eye: The Quest for a new Paradigm*, (Anchor Books, 1983).
Grof, S., *Beyond the Brain* (Suny, 1985).
Grof, S. & Grof,C., *The Stormy Search for the Self*, (Tarcher 1970).
Rowan J. & Dryden, W. (eds), *Innovative Therapy in Britain*, (Open University Press, Milton Keynes, 1988).
Boyne, E. (ed), *Psychotherapy in Ireland*, (Columba Press, Dublin).

APPROACHES

## List of Practitioners

*For addresses and telephone numbers, please refer to the Directory section.*

APPROACHES

ARNOLD, Mavis
ARTHURS, Mary
AYLWIN, Susan
BAILEY, Jane
BEIRNE, Rosarii
BERGIN, Alexander John
BERMINGHAM, Anne Marie
BOGGINS, Tom
BOLAND, Emille
BOYNE, Edward
BREHONY, Rita
BROPHY, Margaret T.M.
BROSNAN, Joan
BROWNE, Larry
BURNS, Maura
BURSTALL, Taru
BUTLER, Maggie
BYRNE, Carmel
BYRNE, Ruth
CALLANAN, Fiodhna
CAMPBELL, Carmel
CANAVAN, Mary
CARROLL, Anna
CLAFFEY, Elaine
CLARKE, Margaret
COLGAN, Patrick J.
COLLEARY, Maura
COLLINS, Barbara
COLLINS, Deirdre
COLLINS-SMYTH, Margaret
CONAGHAN, Mary
CONNOLLY, Brendan M.
CONROY, Kay
COYLE, Brigid
CUNNINGHAM, Kathy
CUNNINGHAM, Nora

CURTIN, Gerardine
DE BURCA, Bairbre
DEERY, Patrick
DENENY, Mary
DEVLIN, Fiona
DIBBLE, Annie
DOYLE, Grainne
DOYLE, Mary
DOYLE, Rosaleen
DRISCOLL, Angela
DUFFY, Kathleen
DUFFY, Martin
DUGGAN, Noël
DULLAGHAN, Elizabeth
   (Lillie)
DUNNE, Ann Maria
DUNNE, Patricia
DWYER, Frankie-Ann
ELLIS, Mary
FAHY, Bernadette
FINLAYSON, Douglas
FITZGERALD, Ann
FITZGERALD, Barbara
FLEMING, Pearl
FLYNN, Madeleine
FLYNN, Stephen
FOLEY, Dermot
FOLEY, Miriam A.
FORDE, Angela
FOX, Michael
FOY, Emma
FRAWLEY, Angela
FRAWLEY, Michael
FULTON, Linda
GILL, Anne
GILMARTIN, Helen

GRIMLEY, Carmel
GRINDLEY, Geraldine M
GUNNE, Dorothy
HARRINGTON, Eileen
HAUGHEY, Monica
HEFFERNAN, Michael
HEGARTY, Owen
HEGARTY, Tony
HERLIHY, Marie
HESKIN, Christina
HILL, Rosemary
HOLLAND, Joanna
HONNAY, Emiel
HORNER, Carol
HOWLETT, Brian G.
HUNTER, Alison I.
JACKSON, Ann
JACKSON, Caitriona
JONES, Coleen
JONES, Helen
JOYCE, Nora
JUDGE, Jimmy
KEHOE, Helen
KELLIHER, Anne
KIERNAN, Donal
KILGALLEN, Aideen
KILLORAN-GANNON,
    Sheila
KILMARTIN, Annie
KLOPP, Marianne
KOHNSTAMM, Barbara
KRZECZUNOWICZ, Sarah
    (Kay)
LANIGAN, Nora
LAWLOR, Mary Brigid
LEWIS, Maeve
LINDEN, Mairead
LINDSAY, John
LINDSAY, Susan

LOGAN, Paddy
LONERGAN, Mary-Anna
LOUGHLIN, Paula
LYNCH, Barbara
LYNCH, Catherine
MACNAMARA, Vincent
MAC NEILL, Sile
MADDEN, Louise
MAGUIRE, Una
MAHER, Ann
MAIR, Bridget
MANGAN, Mary
MANNION WALSHE,
    Deirdre
MARTIN, Ray
MC CABE, Nancy
MC CARTHY, Aine
MC CARTHY, Angela
MC CARTHY, Anne
MC CORMACK, Marijke
MC COURT, Ann
MC COURT, Marie
MC DONNELL, Tricia
MC GEE, Annette
MC LEAVEY, Bernadette
MEAGHER, Kathleen A.
MELVIN, Joan
MERNAGH, Elizabeth
MOHALLY, Derry
MORRISSEY, Germaine
MULLER, Elisabeth
MULLIGAN, Kathleen
MURPHY, David
MURPHY, Ger
MURPHY, Mary
MURRAY, Mary
MYERS, Gerry
NANNERY, Teresa
NEWMAN, Josephine

**APPROACHES**

Ní UALLACHÁIN, Méabh
NOLAN, Inger
NOLAN, Patrick
NORMAND, Tessa
O'BYRNE, Celine
O'CONNOR, Aine
O'CONNOR, Karen E.
O'CONNOR, Marika
O'CONNOR, Mary Rose
O'DEA, Catherine
O'DOHERTY, Colm
O'DONOGHUE, Eilis
O'DONOGHUE, Jim
O'DONOGHUE, Paul
O'DONOVAN, Joan
O'DONOVAN, Margot
O'DOWD, Maura
O'DWYER, Mary
O'FARRELL, Magda
O'GRADY, Bernadette
O'HANLON, Judy
O'LEARY, Eleanor
O'MAHONY, Berenice
O'MAHONY, Hank
O'NEILL, Ann
O'NEILL, Deborah
O'NEILL, Julia
O'NEILL, Mary
O'NEILL, Nora
O'REILLY, Joseph
O'ROURKE, Darina
O'SULLIVAN, Ann
O'SULLIVAN, Rita
O'TOOLE, Muriel
PARKS, Ann
PEAKIN, Anne
PERREM, Breda
PRENDERVILLE, Mary
RIGNEY, Jeanette

RINTOUL, Irene
RIORDAN, Gillian
ROCHE, Anne
ROTHERY, Nuala
RUTH-MURRAY, Ann
RYAN, Anne
RYAN, Anne
RYAN, Catherine
RYAN, David
RYAN, Teresa,
RYAN, Toni
SAHAFI, Janet E.
SAMPSON, Annie
SCULLY, Ros
SELL, Patrick
SHEILL, Mary
SHORTEN, Karen Ilean
SMYTH, Geraldine
SPARROW, Bobbie
STONE, William
SWAIN, Ronny
SWEENEY, Delma
TIERNEY, Maggie
TROOP, Deborah
UNDERWOOD-QUINN,
    Nicola
VAN HOUT, Els
WALLACE, Carmel
WALLACE, George
WALSH, Mary-Paula
WARD, Mary
WARD, Shirley A.
WARDEN, Norman
WATSON, Patricia
WOODS, Jean B.
WRIXON-GOGGIN, Pauline

# Constructivist Psychotherapy (ICPA)

When a person seeks psychotherapy, they have a story to tell. It may be a troubled, hurt or angry story of a life or a relationship now spoiled. For many, it is a story of distressing events which seem to work against a sense of well-being, self confidence, or effectiveness in life. Whatever its form, a therapist is presented with a story, often persuasive and gripping. Of course there are many ways of responding to clients' stories, and different schools of therapy emphasise and engage different aspects of the story. A therapist working from a Constructivist or allied school will, from the outset, realise that a story is more than just a report of a person's experience. They will realise that a story also acts to create, sustain or alter ways in which a client understands and relates to their life circumstances. The therapist will be looking to what kinds of action a particular story invites into a person's life. What kind of understanding and conduct are being engendered, facilitated, or sustained as a result of their particular story. Therapists trained in this School of Psychotherapy will, in general, be concerned to find ways of inviting clients to attend to the manner in which their accounts, those of others, and that of the community in general, act as constraints to more co-operative personal engagements. The emphasis on an invitational approach to ways of making sense of experience is perhaps the clearest hallmark of Constructivist and related schools of therapy.

Expertise in objectivity is relinquished in favour of an invitational exploration of possible ways of accounting and relating to circumstances. Therapists will generally be open to work with individuals, couples, families or wider groups.

For those with an academic or technical interest, some prominent key figures upon which this school of therapy intellectually, historically draws are, Gregory Bateson, George Kelly, David Smail, Miller Mair, W. Barrett Pearce, and Ken Gergen. Locally, key contributors have been Vincent Kenny and Bernadette O'Sullivan.

Some recommended reading would include:

Fay Fransella, *George Kelly*, (Sage Publications, London 1995)

Miller Mair, *Between Psychology and Psychotherapy: A Poetics of Experience*, (Routledge, London 1989)

*Contact address:*   The Secretary, ICPA, 2, Dungar Terrace, Northumberland Road, Dun Laoghaire, Co Dublin. Telephone: (01) 2843336

### List of Practitioners
*For addresses and telephone numbers, please refer to the Directory section.*

| | |
|---|---|
| BAIRD, Jane | LUCEY, Joe |
| BYRNE, Tim | MAGEE, David Louis |
| CAHILL, Michele | MC KEE, Maud |
| COLLINS, Mary | NAUGHTON, Annemarie |
| DALY, Margaret | NOLAN, Bernadette |
| DAVEY, Damien | O'BRIEN, Gay |
| DELMONTE, M. M. | O'DONNELL, Godfrey |
| EGAN, Barbara | O'SULLIVAN, Bernadette |
| FLYNN, Deirdre | RUSSELL, Maura |
| FOLEY, Robert | SWEENEY, Brion |
| GALLIGAN, Patricia | VAN DOORSLAER, Mia |
| GUNNE, David | WADE, Richard A. |
| GUNNE, Dorothy | WALSH, Mary-Paula |
| KENNY, Vincent | WALSH, Tony |

APPROACHES

## Psychoanalytic Psychotherapy

The three sub-divisions within this section are:
1. IFCAPP
2. IFPP
3. IGAS

### Child and Adolescent Psychoanalytic Psychotherapy (IFCAPP)

Child and Adolescent Psychoanalytic Psychotherapy is a relatively new discipline in Ireland, although it has been practised widely in Europe and North America for fifty years. Most therapists working with children in Ireland have been trained under the auspices of the Irish Forum for Child and Adolescent Psychoanalytic Psychotherapy and Trinity College, Dublin. This therapy aims at helping children and adolescents learn a greater degree of self-understanding in the setting of a secure therapeutic relationship. Children are helped to learn, not only self awareness, but also how their pattern of relationships has been formed and how this may influence present experiences. Children in therapy are also afforded the opportunity to experience a new type of relationship in a safe, therapeutic setting. Such therapy can happen through a mixture of talk, play and activity.

*Contact address:*  The Secretary, IFCAPP,
13, Stradbrook Lawn,
Blackrock, Co Dublin
Telephone: (01) 2806623

### The Irish Forum for Psychoanalytic Psychotherapy (IFPP)

Members of the Irish Forum for Psychoanalytic Psychotherapy (IFPP) are professional psychotherapists who come from the different schools of psychoanalytic thought which originated with Freud in the late 19th century. Psychoanalytic Psychotherapy involves uncovering unconscious conflicts and causes of distress and elucidating desires both conscious and unconscious by means of free association, exploration of dream material, feelings and memories. The working through of this material brings alive both the past and the present.

The Irish Forum for Psychoanalytic Psychotherapy was founded in 1986 with the aim of providing coherent focus for those people throughout the island with a serious interest in the advancement of the study and practice of psychoanalytic psychotherapy, which remains central to the organisation today. All full members of the IFPP have fulfilled training requirements which are in line with colleagues in the rest of Europe.

*Contact address:* Martin Boyle, IFPP,
St Saviour's, Dorset Street, Dublin 1.
Tel: (01) 4513076 / 087-2845637

### Group Analysis (IGAS)

Group Analysis is a method of group psychotherapy which was initiated in 1940 in England by the late Dr. S. H. Foulkes and has since been refined and developed by an ever widening circle of associates of practitioners, both in England and abroad.

### Irish Context

In 1987, the Institute of Group Analysis London, in association with the School of Psychotherapy St Vincent's Hospital and University College Dublin, established the Group Analytic Psychotherapy Training in Ireland. The first Group Analysts graduated in 1994 and at present, there are 60 trainees at varying stages in the training programme. In the Spring of 1996, the newly formed Irish Group Analytic

Society ran its first Public Workshop in Dublin entitled 'Loss, Change and Creativity'. The workshop succeeded very well in its aim, which offered an opportunity for people working with Groups, and for individuals, to gain an experience of Group Analysis through working with this particular theme which has such important personal and social implications for Ireland at the present time.

### What is Group Analysis?

Group Analysis is primarily a method of group psychotherapy which combines psychoanalytic insights with an understanding of social and interpersonal factors. It focuses on the relationship between the individual and the group in order to strengthen the development of both. The ultimate aim is to achieve the integration of the individual in his or her communal network, which is the hallmark of a healthy society. Its orientation is analytic, deriving from the principles of psychoanalysis, but differing from psychoanalysis in the light of certain important concepts that have been arrived at by considering the individual member in the context of the group as a whole. Group Analysis focuses on the dynamics within the group between all its members, including the therapist.

### How does it work?

In practice, the small analytic group consists of not more than eight members and the analyst. Members will not be known to each other before joining the group, and social contact outside the group is discouraged. The groups will contain both men and women and members will join for a variety of reasons. Confidentiality is of the utmost importance. The group will usually meet once or twice a week at the same time and in the same place for a duration of one and a half hours, and all the business of the group is conducted and contained within this time. This type of group will continue to exist for many years, and the membership will change as the individuals are ready to leave and new members join. The analyst will assess each individual member, and there will be a short period of preparation, before joining the group. The process of change is a slow process and for a member to get maximum benefit from the group therapeutic situation, members would stay for about two years minimum. Most analysts work on a sliding scale, and usually each session costs approximately £15.

### Applied Group Analysis

Group Analytic Psychotherapy is also widely applied in the work setting with staff and with small and large working groups, and with psychological problems with children, adolescents, couples and the elderly. Other areas of therapeutic application include: learning disabilities, psychosexual and psychosomatic problems, alcohol and drug dependence, eating, mood and personality disorders, psychosis and long-term mental illness. The three main groups in which group analytic psychotherapy is practised, are the small group (as described above), the medium group (more than 10 and less than 25) and the large group (more than 25 and upwards).

### The Core Professions

The core professions of the Group Analysts include Psychiatrists, Psychologists, Social Workers, Nurses, Counsellors, Teachers, Clergy/Religious and Occupational Therapists. The Group Analysts work both in the Private and the Public Sectors.

*Contact Address:*　　IGAS,
　　　　　　　　　　　Global House,
　　　　　　　　　　　29 Lower Abbey Street, Dublin 1.
　　　　　　　　　　　Tel: (01) 8786486

## List of Practitioners

*For addresses and telephone numbers, please refer to the Directory section.*

### IFCAPP

ANDREWS, Paul
BEAUMONT, Margaret
BREEN, Noreen
BREEN, Thomas
CASEY, Grainne
CONNOLLY, Margaret
DILLON, Marie T.
DONNELLY, Patricia
DOYLE, Sherry
FORBES, Jean
HARGIN, Mary Rose
JEFFRIES, Mary
MURPHY, Zoe
NEARY, Nora
NÍ GHALLCHOBHAIR,
 Maighread
NIC DHOMHNAILL, Caoimhe
O'CONNELL, Patricia
O'FLAHERTY, Anne
O'GRADY, Paul
O'HORA, Claire
O'SULLIVAN, Marych
OWENS, Conor
PHALAN, Sally
WIECZOREK-DEERING, Dorit.

### IFPP

BOYLE, Martin
BRENT, Rebecca
BRIGHT, Jill
BUCKLEY, Marion
CASSERLY, Felicity
CHILDERS, Nessa
COLEMAN, Padraig
COX, Ann
COX CAMERON, Olga
CULLEN, Mary
DALY, Martin J.

DELMONTE, M.M.
DONOGHUE, Mary
DUNLEA, Marian
EGAN, Angela
FRENCH, Gerry
GLEESON, Betty
GRIEVE, Karin
GROVER, Mary
JENNINGS, Norman
KEARNEY, Ruth
MAHER, Bonnie
MASTERSON, Ingrid
MC CARRICK, Tom
MC CARTHY, Rita
MURPHY, Ann
MURPHY, Brendan
NI NUALLAIN, Mairin
NOLAN, Patrick
NOWLAN, Kate
O'MAHONY, Catherine
O'MALLEY-DUNLOP, Ellen
O'SULLIVAN, Marych
PYLE, Mary
RYAN, Derval
SHEEHAN, Mary
SKAR, Patricia
SKELTON, Ross
SWEENEY, Irene M.
WEATHERILL, Rob
WILSDON, Sheelagh
YOUNG, Anne

### IGAS

BENSON, Jarlath F
BERMINGHAM, Paula
COGHLAN, Helena
DEENY, Peggy
DOWD, Teresa
DUNCAN, Audrey

APPROACHES

FAHY, Michael
FINNEGAN, Leo
GARLAND, Clive
O'BRIEN, David

O'MALLEY-DUNLOP, Ellen
RYAN, Derval
SMITH, Ray
SOMERS, Olive

APPROACHES

# PART III

# A Directory
## of Psychotherapists in Ireland

**ANDREWS, Paul**
36 Lower Leeson Street, Dublin 2.
Tel: 01-6767321
IFCAPP

**ARNOLD, Mavis**
Rosney Mews, Albert Road,
Glenageary, Co Dublin.
Tel: 01-2805575
IAHIP

**ARTHURS, Mary**
Dubhlinn Institute,
16 Prospect Road,
Glasnevin, Dublin 9.
Tel: 01 - 8302358
IAHIP

**AYLWIN, Susan**
Dept. of Applied Psychology,
University College,
Cork.
Tel: 021-902368
IAHIP

**BAILEY, Jane**
Clondalkin Addiction Support
Programme, Ballyowen Meadows,
Fonthill Road,
Clondalkin, Dublin 22.
*and* Loreto Centre,
Crumlin Road, Dublin 12
Tel: 01-6238030/4535048/
087-2922584
IAHIP

**BAIRD, Jane**
11, The Green, Beaumont Woods,
Beaumont, Dublin 9.
Tel: 01-8379191/087-2323601
ICPA

**BANNON, John**
St Fintan's Hospital,
Portlaoise, Co Laois.
Tel: 0502 - 21364
FTAI

**BARRY, Kathleen**
Mental Health Centre,
Markievicz House,
Barrack Street, Sligo.
Tel: 071-55120
CBT

**BAYLY, Kathrin**
29, College Park Way,
Dublin 16
Tel: 01-2960803
FTAI

**BEAUMONT, Margaret**
Strand Road, Merrion,
Dublin 4
Tel: 01-2693951
IFCAPP

BEIRNE, Rosarii
Lanesboro, Co Longford
Tel: 087-2331011
IAHIP

BENNETT, Eamonn
Loughanstown, Knockdrin,
Mullingar, Co Westmeath
Tel: 044-71251
CBT

BENSON, Jarlath F.
10 Mill Road, Drumaness,
Ballynahinch, Co Down BT24 8SF
Tel: 01238-564420
IGAS

BERGIN, Alexander John
6 Patrick Street,
Mountmellick, Co Laois.
Tel: 0502-24299
IAHIP

BERMINGHAM, Anne Marie
Huntersmoon, Sydenham Villas,
Dundrum, Dublin 14.
Tel: 01-2980567
IAHIP

BERMINGHAM, Paula
63 Kimmage Grove, Dublin 6W.
Tel: 01- 4908315
IGAS

BOGGINS, Tom
414 Ard Mhuire,
Rathangan, Co Kildare
Tel: 045-524893
IAHIP

BOLAND, Emille
206 Moyville,
Rathfarnham, Dublin 16.
Tel: 01-4945818
IAHIP

BOURKE, Carmel
St Anne's Secondary School,
Tipperary Town,
Co Tipperary.
Tel: 062-51747
FTAI

BOYLE, Martin
St Saviour's, Dorset Street,,
Dublin 1.
Tel: 087-2845637/4513076
IFPP

BOYNE, Edward
24 Clarinda Park East,
Dun Laoghaire, Co Dublin.
Tel: 01-2809178
IAHIP

BREEN, Noreen
CDVEC Psychological Service,
25 Temple Road,
Dartry, Dublin 6.
Tel: 01 -4971442
IFCAPP

BREEN, Thomas
St Joseph's Adolescent & Family
Service,
193 Richmond Road,
Fairview, Dublin 3
Tel: 01-8842430
IFCAPP

BREHONY, Rita
18 Glenard Ave,
Salthill, Galway.
Tel: 091-522648
IAHIP

BRENT, Rebecca
Roscahill Pier, Kilmeena,
Westport, Co Mayo
Tel: 098-41914
IFPP

BRIGHT, Jill
2 Alexandra Place,
St Luke's,
Cork.
Tel: 021-507360
IFPP

BROPHY, Margaret T. M.
No 1 Leo Street, Dublin 7.
Tel: 088-2128414
IAHIP

BROPHY, John
Marino, Dublin 3.
Tel: 01-8338615
FTAI

BROSNAN, Joan
18 Hazelwood, Taylor's Hill,
Galway
Tel: 091-529057
IAHIP

BROWNE, Essie,
Psychiatric Unit,
Cavan General Hospital, Cavan.
Tel: 049-4361399
FTAI

BROWNE, Larry
69 Greenwood Estate, Glasheen Rd,
Cork.
Tel: 021-963511/087-2026751
IAHIP

BUCKLEY, Marion
18 Carton Court, Maynooth,
Co Kildare
Tel: 01-6286676
IFPP

BUCKLEY, Marguerite
Galway Diocesan Pastoral Centre,
Arus de Brun,
Newtownsmith, Galway.
Tel: 091-65066
FTAI

BURBRIDGE, Paul
St Davnet's Hospital, Monaghan
Tel: 047-81822
CBT

BURKE, Phil
St Vincent's Hospital,
Richmond Road, Fairview,
Dublin 3
Tel: 01-8375101 / 087-2442325
CBT

BURNS, Maura
Wave Trauma Centre
Tel: 01232 779922
IAHIP

BURSTALL, Taru
11 North Terrace,
Inchicore, Dublin 8.
Tel: 01-4733819
IAHIP

BUTLER, Goretti
Management Office,
14 Baggot Road,
Navan Road, Dublin 7.
Tel: 01-8686050/8680681
FTAI

BUTLER, Maggie
Vico Consultation Centre,
2 Dungar Terrace, Dun Laoghaire,
Co Dublin.
Tel: 01-2843336/087-2607258
IAHIP

**BYRNE, Carmel**
'Amethyst', 28 Beechcourt,
Killiney, Co Dublin.
Tel: 01-2850976
IAHIP

**BYRNE, Nollaig**
Mater Hospital,
Dublin
Tel: 01-8034793
FTAI

**BYRNE, Patrick**
Tralee General Hospital,
Tralee, Co Kerry.
Tel: 066-7126222
FTAI

**BYRNE, Ruth**
Coolagh,
Dungarvan, Co Waterford.
Tel: 058-43057
IAHIP

**BYRNE, Tim**
Ballamona Hospital,
Strang, Isle of Man
Tel: 01624 642 642
ICPA

**CADWELL, Nuala**
Connect Associates,
Lonsdale House, Avoca Road,
Blackrock, Co Dublin.
Tel: 01-2884155
FTAI/IAHIP

**CAHILL, Michele**
Naas General Hospital,
Tús Nua, Dublin Road,
Kildare, Co Kildare
Tel: 045-521220/01-2603183
ICPA

**CALLANAN, Fiodhna**
Dublin Rape Crisis Centre,
70 Lr Leeson St., Dublin 2.
Tel: 01-6774911
IAHIP

**CALLANAN, William**
Milltown Park,
Sandford Road, Dublin 6.
Tel: 01-2698411
FTAI

**CAMPBELL, Carmel**
15 Forest Walk, River Valley,
Swords, Co Dublin
Tel: 01-8407984
IAHIP

**CANAVAN, Mary**
'Avalon', 8 Alma Park,
Monkstown Village, Co Dublin.
Tel: 01-2845208
IAHIP

**CARBERRY, Brian**
Hampton Health Centre,
Hampton Street,
Balbriggan, Co Dublin.
Tel: 01-8413930/1
FTAI

**CARR, Alan**
Dept of Psychology, UCD,
Room 232, Science Building,
Belfield, Dublin 4.
Tel: 01-7062390/7062123
FTAI

**CARROLL, Anna**
Eckhart House,
19 Clyde Road, Dublin 4
Tel: 01-6684687
IAHIP

CARROLL, Patricia
Clanwilliam Institute,
18 Clanwilliam Tce, Dublin 2 *and*
Shankill, *and* Newtown-
mountkennedy, Co Wicklow.
Tel: 01-2873162/6761363
FTAI

CARTON, Simone
National Brain Injury Service,
National Rehabilitation Hospital,
Rochestown Avenue,
Dun Laoghaire, Co Dublin.
Tel: 01-2854777
FTAI

CASEY, Grainne
Arduna, 54 Clontarf Road,
Dublin 3.
Tel: 01-8332733
IFCAPP

CASSERLY, Felicity
Blackrock, Co Dublin.
Tel: 01-2882286
IFPP

CHILDERS, Nessa
14 Gledswood Avenue,
Clonskeagh, Dublin 14.
Tel: 01-2697682
IFPP

CLAFFEY, Elaine
4 Pembroke Cottages,
Dundrum, Dublin 14.
Tel: 01-2962115
IAHIP

CLARKE, Margaret
23 Lr. Albert Road,
Sandycove, Co Dublin.
Tel: 01-2808989
IAHIP

CLARKE, Michele
Social Services Inspectorate,
c/o Hawkins House, Dublin 2
Tel: 01-4922209
FTAI

COGHLAN, Helena
41 Lower Baggot Street,
Dublin 2.
Tel: 01-6609490
IGAS

COLEMAN, Padraig
27 Fitzwilliam Square, Dublin 2.
Tel: 01-6761626
IFPP

COLGAN, Patrick J.
Inst. of Psychosynthesis &
Transpersonal Theory,
Eckhart House,
19 Clyde Road, Dublin 4.
Tel: 01-6684687
IAHIP

COLLEARY, Maura
Eckhart House,
19 Clyde Road, Dublin 4.
Tel: 01-2844256
IAHIP

COLLINS, Barbara
New Day Counselling Centre,
Dublin
Tel: 01-8453474
IAHIP

COLLINS, Deirdre
Dundrum Counselling & Therapy
Centre, 4 Pembroke Cottages,
Pye Centre, Dundrum, Dublin 14
Tel: 01-4937394
IAHIP

COLLINS, Mary
Plezicia House,
Dunlavin, Co Wicklow
Tel: 045-401725
ICPA

COLLINS, Geraldine
Shannon Health Centre,
Mid Western Health Board,
Shannon, Co Clare.
Tel: 061-362491/362459
FTAI

COLLINS, Ines
Clanwilliam Institute,
18 Clanwilliam Terrace,
Grand Canal Quay, Dublin 2.
Tel: 01-6761363/6762881
FTAI

COLLINS-SMYTH, Margaret
'Mignon',
Corbally Road, Limerick.
Tel: 061-347506
IAHIP

CONAGHAN, Mary
18 Casimir Road,
Harold's Cross, Dublin 6W.
Tel: 01-4908883
IAHIP

CONNEELY, Caitlin
5 College Crescent, The Pines,
Ballinasloe, Co Galway
Tel: 0905-45202
FTAI

CONNOLLY, Brendan
Moore Abbey,
Monasterevin, Co Kildare.
Tel: 045-525327
FTAI

CONNOLLY, Brendan M.
7 Brookville Estate,
Glanmire, Co Cork.
Tel: 021-821774
IAHIP

CONNOLLY, Margaret
24 Dornden Park, Booterstown,
Co Dublin
Tel: 01-2838441
IFCAPP

CONROY, Kay
Turning Point, 23 Crofton Road,
Dun Laoghaire, Co Dublin.
Tel: 01-2801094
IAHIP

COSTELLO, Margaret T.
Child & Family Centre,
St Mary's, Dublin Road,
Drogheda, Co. Louth.
Tel: 041-9830990
FTAI

COX, Ann
Arduna, 54 Clontarf Road,
Dublin 3.
Tel: 01-8332733
IFPP

COX CAMERON, Olga
19 Belgrave Square,
Monkstown, Co Dublin.
Tel: 01-2808868
IFPP

COYLE, Brigid
100, St Lawrence Road,
Clontarf, Dublin 3
Tel: 01-8332479
IAHIP

CULLEN, Mary
Frascati Park,
Blackrock, Co Dublin
Tel: 01-2831532
IFPP

CUNNINGHAM, Kathy
Holy Spirit Convent,
Mallow, Co Cork
Tel: 022-21780
IAHIP

CUNNINGHAM, Nora
Dirreen, Athea,
Co Limerick.
Tel: 068-42232
IAHIP

CURTIN, Gerardine
Markievicz House,
Sligo.
Tel: 071-44029
IAHIP

DALY, Margaret,
Dept of Psychology,UCD,
Belfield, Dublin 4
Tel: 01-7068612
ICPA

DALY, Martin
89 Lr. Leeson Street,
Dublin 2.
Tl: 01-6762586
FTAI

DALY, Martin J.
2 Church Lane,
Lr. Kilmacud Road, Co Dublin.
Tel: 01-2882257
IFPP

DAVEY, Damien
199 Fitzwilliam Terrace,
Lr Dartry Road, Dublin 6.
Tel: 01-4978476
ICPA

DE BURCA, Bairbre
Eckhart House,
19, Clyde Road, Dublin 4.
Tel: 01-6684687
IAHIP

DE JONGH, Corry
Clanwilliam Institute,
18 Clanwilliam Terrace,
Dublin 2.
Tel: 01-6761363/6762881
FTAI

DE LACY, Mara
St Patrick's Hospital,
James' Street, Dublin 8.
Tel: 01-6775423
FTAI

DEENY, Peggy
Mourneside Medical Centre,
Strabane Co Tyrone *and*
Showfield, Stranorlar, Co Donegal.
Tel: 01504-351374 / 074-32746
IGAS

DEERY, Patrick
104 Muirhevna, Dublin Road,
Dundalk, Co Louth.
Tel: 042-9331848
IAHIP

DELAHUNTY, Alan
The Medical Centre, 6 Snipe Lawn,
Newcastle, Co Galway
Tel: 087-2309037/091-521666
FTAI

## DELMONTE, M. M.
St Patrick's Hospital,
James' Street, Dublin 8.
Tel: 01-6775423 (W) / 2804477 (H)
IFPP & ICPA

## DENENY, Mary
5 The Elms, Forster Street,
Galway.
Tel: 087-2624023
IAHIP

## DENNEHY, Noreen
Clanwilliam Institute,
18 Clanwilliam Terrace,
Grand Canal Quay, Dublin 2.
Tel: 01- 6761363/6762881
FTAI

## DEVLIN, Fiona
6, Sydney Place,
Wellington Road, Cork.
Tel: 021-507247
IAHIP

## DEVLIN, Teresa
Millbrae Surgery,
Millbrae, Carndonagh, Co Donegal.
Tel: 077-74644/74214
CBT

## DIBBLE, Annie
56, Inchicore Road,
Dublin 8.
Tel: 01-4537304
IAHIP

## DILLON, Marie T.
Lucena Clinic, Orwell Road, Rathgar
and Churchtown Medical Centre,
69, Upr Churchtown Road,
Churchtown, Dublin 14.
Tel: 01-2981801
IFCAPP

## DOCKERY, Bernadette
167, Lr Drumcondra Road,
Drumcondra, Dublin 9.
Tel: 01-8371336
FTAI

## DOHERTY, Myra
Day Centre,
The Rock,
Ballymote, Co Sligo.
Tel: 071-83002
CBT

## DONNELLY, Patricia
Barnardos, Christchurch Square,
Dublin 8.
Tel: 01-4530355(W)/2864053(H)
IFCAPP

## DONOGHUE, Mary
17 Seapoint Avenue,
Blackrock, Co Dublin
Tel: 01-2808177
IFPP

## DOOLEY, Deirdre
Hesed House, 74 Tyrconnell Road,
Inchicore, Dublin 8.
Tel: 01-4549474
FTAI

## DOWD, Teresa
St Camillus Unit,
St Vincent's Hospital,
Elm Park, Dublin 4.
Tel: 01-2094577
IGAS

## DOWNEY, Betty
4 Chapel Street,
Carrick-on-Suir, Co Tipperary
Tel: 051-641346
FTAI

DOYLE, Grainne
30, Ashbrook Park,
Ennis Road, Limerick
Tel: 061-452224
IAHIP

DOYLE, Mary
16 Salmon View Terrace,
Sunday's Well Avenue, Cork.
Tel: 021-301187
IAHIP

DOYLE, Rosaleen
Inst. of Psychosynthesis &
Transpersonal Theory,
Eckhart House,
19 Clyde Road, Dublin 4.
Tel: 01-6684687
IAHIP

DOYLE, Sherry
Milltown Medical Centre,
98 Lower Churchtown Road,
Dublin 14.
Tel: 01-2960918
IFCAPP

DRISCOLL, Angela
Front Garden Flat,
43 Alma Road,
Monkstown, Co Dublin.
Tel: 01-2843172
IAHIP

DRISCOLL, Zelie
44 Lr. Newcastle, Galway.
Tel: 091-791087
FTAI

DUFFY, Kathleen
Westport Road,
Castlebar, Co Mayo.
Tel: 094-24206
IAHIP

DUFFY, Martin
Dunderry Park Transpersonal Ctr.,
Dunderry, Navan, Co Meath.
Tel: 046-74455
IAHIP

DUFFY, Mary
Glenmalure Day Hospital,
Milltown Road, Dublin 6.
Tel: 01-2830388
FTAI

DUGGAN, Colman
157 Delwood Close,
Castleknock, Dublin 15.
Tel: 01-8212845
FTAI

DUGGAN, Noël
3, Greenview Heights,
Inishannagh Park,
Newcastle, Galway.
Tel: 091-526126
IAHIP

DULLAGHAN, Elizabeth
(Lillie)
'Oakdene', 3 Seatown Place,
Dundalk, Co Louth.
Tel: 042-9338333 (W) 9333674 (H)
IAHIP

DUNCAN, Audrey
The Medical Centre, Mary Street,
Clonmel, Co Tipperary
Tel: 052-21288/25236
IGAS

DUNLEA, Marian
19, Trafalgar Terrace,
Monkstown, Co. Dublin
Tel: 01-2800572
IFPP

### DUNNE, Ann Maria
Chrysalis Holistic Centre,
Donard, Co Wicklow.
Tel: 045-404713
IAHIP

### DUNNE, Patricia
Dundalk, Co Louth.
Tel: 042-9371976
IAHIP

### DWYER, Frankie-Ann
9 Albany Road,
Ranelagh, Dublin 6.
Tel: 01-4973425
IAHIP

### EGAN, Angela
124, Ranelagh, Dublin 6
Tel: 01-4962595
IFPP

### EGAN, Barbara
Fortlands, 5, Meath Road,
Bray, Co. Wicklow
Tel: 01-2762391
ICPA

### ELLIS, Mary
1 The Crescent,
Cobh, Co Cork.
Tel: 021-811679
IAHIP

### FADDEN, Rosaleen
Ionad Follain,
Myshall, Co Carlow.
Tel: 0503-57810
FTAI

### FAHY, Bernadette,
25 Longford Terrace,
Dun Laoghaire, Co Dublin
Tel: 01-2860298
IAHIP

### FAHY, Michael
Galway Group Analytic Psychotherapy
Practice, Prospect House,
Prospect Hill, Galway.
Tel: 091-567344
IGAS

### FAY, Joe
Probation & Welfare Service,
Smithfield Chambers,
Dublin 7.
Tel: 01-8173600
FTAI

### FINGLETON, May
1 Fitzmaurice Place,
Portlaoise, Co Laois and
Friary Court Family Therapy Svcs,
Friary Street, Kilkenny
Tel: 0502-27176/ 087-2310008
FTAI

### FINLAYSON, Douglas
2 Alexandra Place,
St Lukes, Cork.
Tel: 021-500307
IAHIP

### FINNEGAN, Leo J.
Human Development & Relations
Practice, Glencar Scotch,
Letterkenny, Co Donegal.
Tel: 074-26405
IGAS

### FITZGERALD, Ann
Mahareese,
Castlegregory, Co Kerry
Tel: 066-7139370
IAHIP

### FITZGERALD, Barbara
Eckhart House,
19 Clyde Road,
Ballsbridge, Dublin 4.
Tel: 01-2894787
IAHIP & FTAI

## FITZMAURICE, John
1A Beatty Grove,
Celbridge, Co Kildare
Tel: 01-6271010/086-2397940
CBT

## FLEMING, Pearl
4 Pembroke Cottages,
PYE Centre, Ballinteer Road,
Dundrum, Dublin 14.
Tel: 01-2962115
IAHIP

## FLYNN, Deirdre
Student Counselling Service,
House 6, Trinity College,
Dublin
Tel: 01-6081407 (W)
ICPA

## FLYNN, Madeleine
15C Sandycove Ave East,
Sandycove, Co Dublin
Tel: 01-2805577.
IAHIP

## FLYNN, Stephen
Sangrail Healing Practice,
c/o Hickey, Fitzgerald O'Brien St.,
Mallow, Co Cork.
Tel: 087-2870100
IAHIP

## FOLEY, Dermot
21, Leeson Park, Dublin 6
Tel: 01-2600773
IAHIP

## FOLEY, Miriam A.
'Ambeldene', The Mullagh,
Kilcock, Co Meath
Tel: 01-6289164
IAHIP

## FOLEY, Robert
2, Eden Park,
Dun Laoghaire, Co. Dublin
Tel: 01-2800084
ICPA

## FORBES, Jean
Dept of Child & Family Psychiatry,
Mater Hospital, NCR, Dublin 7
*and* Arduna,
53 Clontarf Road, Dublin 3.
Tel: 01-8032516
IFCAPP

## FORDE, Angela
Knock Shrine,
Knock, Co Mayo.
Tel: 094-88100
IAHIP

## FORREST, Mary
Teen Counselling,
37 Greenfort Gardens, Dublin
Tel: 01-6231398
FTAI

## FOX, Michael
12 Wainsfort Drive,
Terenure, Dublin 6W.
Tel: 01-4906796
IAHIP

## FOY, Emma
The Mews, Summerhill House,
Marino Avenue West,
Killiney, Co Dublin.
Tel: 01-2840501
IAHIP

## FRASER, Teresa
7 Lisfennel Close,
Dungarvan, Co Waterford.
Tel: 058-43191
FTAI

**FRAWLEY, Angela**
Stepping Stones,
Ballybane Road, Galway.
Tel: 091-755998
IAHIP

**FRAWLEY, Michael**
Stepping Stones,
Ballybane Road, Galway.
Tel: 091-755998
IAHIP

**FRENCH, Gerry**
St Columban's, Navan
and
Mossbrook,
Claremorris, Co Mayo
Tel:046-21525/094-65155
IFPP

**FRYER, Anthony**
7 Church Street,
Youghal, Co Cork
Tel: 024-90166
FTAI

**FULTON, Linda**
46 Elmwood Avenue Lr.,
Ranelagh, Dublin 6.
Tel: 01-4971188/4971722
FTAI/IAHIP

**GAFFNEY, Delia**
Lucena Clinic, Blessington Road,
Tallaght, Dublin 24.
Tel: 01-4526333
FTAI

**GALLIGAN, Claire**
25 Aisling Heights,
Blanchardstown, Dublin 15
Tel: 01-8206170/087-6394897
FTAI

**GALLIGAN, Patricia**
St Vincent's Hospital,
Richmond Road,
Fairview, Dublin 3.
Tel: 01-8375101
ICPA/FTAI

**GARLAND, Clive**
Clanwilliam Institute,
18 Clanwilliam Terrace,
Grand Canal Quay, Dublin 2.
Tel: 01-6761363
IGAS

**GILL, Anne**
6 Windsor Terrace,
Malahide, Co Dublin.
Tel: 01-8450698
IAHIP

**GILLILAND, Kay P.**
7 Beaver Row,
Donnybrook, Dublin 4.
Tel: 01-2691716
FTAI

**GILMARTIN, Helen**
17 Farrenboley Park,
Dundrum, Dublin 14.
Tel: 01-2951210
IAHIP

**GLEESON, Betty**
St Patrick's Hospital,
James's Street, Dublin 8.
Tel: 01-6775423 Ext 431
IFPP/FTAI

**GORDON, Evelyn**
Family Therapy Department,
St Joseph's Adolescent & Family
Services,
193 Richmond Road,
Fairview, Dublin 3
Tel: 01-8842421
FTAI

GRIEVE, Karen
65 Lower Salthill,
Galway.
Tel: 091-521059
IFPP

GRIMLEY, Carmel
2 Manor Rise,
Grange Road, Dublin 16.
Tel: 01-4944441
IAHIP

GRINDLEY, Geraldine M.
33 Brookwood Heights,
Artane, Dublin 5.
Tel: 01-8328016
IAHIP

GROSSMAN FREYNE, Gail
Family Therapy & Counselling Ctr,
46 Elmwood Avenue Lr,
Ranelagh Village, Dublin 6.
Tel: 01-4971188
FTAI

GROVER, Mary
Ardralla, Church Cross,
Skibbereen, Co Cork.
Tel: 028-38373
IFPP

GUNNE, David
St Columba's Hospital,
Sligo
Tel: 074-42111
ICPA

GUNNE, Dorothy
National Training &
Development Institute,
Roslyn Park, Beach Road,
Sandymount, Dublin 4.
Tel: 01-2057344
FTAI/ICPA/IAHIP

HARGIN, Mary Rose
Blackrock, Co Dublin,
Celbridge; Naas, Co Kildare
Tel: 045-869261/087-2200948
IFCAPP

HARNEY, Vivian
Employee Assistance Svc,
Dept of Finance, Room 3.21,
Frederick Buildings,
Sth Frederick St., Dublin 2.
Tel: 01-6798223
CBT

HARRINGTON, Eileen
11 Silverwood,
Ballinlough, Cork.
Tel: 021-295424
IAHIP

HAUGHEY, Monica
31 Cherryfield Avenue,
Ranelgah, Dublin 6.
Tel: 01-4977067
IAHIP

HAYES, Fran
Laragh Counselling Service,
140 St. Lawrence's Road,
Clontarf, Dublin 3.
Tel: 01-8335044
FTAI

HEFFERNAN, Michael
Marino Institute of Education,
Griffith Avenue, Dublin 9.
Tel: 01-8335111
IAHIP

HEGARTY, Donal
Strand House, 3 Phillipsburgh Avenue,
Fairview, Dublin 3
Tel: 01-8369899
FTAI

DIRECTORY

## HEGARTY, Owen
Mercers Health Centre,
Lower Stephen Street, Dublin 2.
Tel: 01-4022307/086-8141177
IAHIP

## HEGARTY, Tony
'Cluainlee', Tower,
Blarney, Co Cork
Tel: 021-383010
IAHIP

## HENNIGAN, Cecily
Family Care Centre,
Cherryorchard Avenue,
Ballyfermot, Dublin
Tel: 01-6231313
FTAI

## HERLIHY, Marie
7 Brookville Estate,
Glanmire, Co Cork.
Tel: 021-821774
IAHIP

## HESKIN, Christina
'Bethesda', Mall House,
Tuam, Co Galway.
Tel: 093-28300
IAHIP

## HILL, Rosemary
Gorey Health Centre,
Hospital Grounds,
Gorey, Co Wexford.
Tel: 055-21374
IAHIP

## HIRST, Iain J.
Markievicz House,
Barracks Street, Sligo.
Tel: 071-55100 Ext 5224
FTAI

## HOLLAND, Joanna
Rock Castle, Kilmacsimon,
Bandon, Co Cork *and*
Suite 3b, Sth Terrace Medical Centre,
South Terrace Court, Cork
Tel: 021-775324
IAHIP

## HOLLAND, Mary
St Joseph's Adolescent &
Family Services,
St Vincent's Hospital,
Richmond Road,
Fairview, Dublin 3.
Tel: 01-8842404
FTAI

## HONNAY, Emiel
13 Beechmount Ave, Navan, Co Meath
*and* Dublin Counselling & Therapy
Centre,
41 Upr Gardiner Street, Dublin 1.
Tel: 046-74019/01-8788236
IAHIP

## HORNER, Carol
21 Wandsworth Road,
Belfast BT4 3LS
Northern Ireland.
Tel: 01232-653651
IAHIP

## HORNER, Philomena
26 Woodville St., Lurgan,
Co Armagh, BT67 9DQ
Tel: 01762-348602(H)
01762-347222(W)
FTAI

## HOULIHAN, Tom
St Vincent's Psychiatric Hospital,
Richmond Rd, Fairview, Dublin 3.
Tel: 01-8375101
FTAI

## HOWARD, Leslie
Acorn Counselling Centre,
Wellington Quay,
Drogheda, Co Louth
Tel: 041-9844277/087-2240309
FTAI

## HOWLETT, Brian G.
Dublin Counselling & Therapy
Centre,
41 Upr Gardiner Street, Dublin 1.
Tel: 01-8788236
IAHIP

## HUNTER, Alison I.
Amethyst, Ballybroghan,
Killaloe, Co. Clare
Tel: 061-376331
IAHIP

## JACKSON, Ann
The Surgery, Bridge House,
Carrigaline, Co Cork
Tel: 021-372663
IAHIP

## JACKSON, Caitriona
Aistear, Gort, Co Galway, *and*
Avoca Avenue. Blackrock,
Co Dublin
Tel: 091-630163/086-8430529
IAHIP

## JEBB, Winston
Teen Counselling,
37 Greenfort Gardens,
Quarryvale,Clondalkin, Dublin 22.
Tel: 01-6231398
FTAI

## JEFFRIES, Mary
St Paul's Hospital & Special School,
Beaumont, Dublin 9
Tel: 01-8377673/8378260
IFCAPP

## JENNINGS, Norman
St John of God Hospital,
Stillorgan, Co Dublin.
Tel: 01-2881781 Ext. 311,
IFPP

## JONES, Coleen
Suite 2, South Terrace Medical Centre,
Infirmary Road, Cork.
Tel: 021-813285
IAHIP

## JONES, Helen
ICCP,
82 Upper Georges Street,
Dun Laoghaire, Co Dublin.
Tel: 01-2802523
IAHIP

## JOYCE, Nora
The Healing House,
24  O'Connell Avenue,
Berkeley Road,  Dublin 7.
Tel: 01-4964940
IAHIP

## JUDGE, Jimmy
New Day Counselling Centre,
11 Meath Street, Dublin 8.
Tel: 01-4547050(W) 087-2852255(H)
IAHIP

## JUTHAN, Kay
53 Grange Road,
Rathfarnham, Dublin 14.
Tel: 01-4947462
FTAI

## KEANE, Verena
Clanwilliam Institute,
18 Clanwilliam Terrace, Dublin 2.
Tel: 01-6761363
FTAI

**KEARNEY, Philip**
Clanwilliam Institute,
18 Clanwilliam Terrace, Dublin 2.
Tel: 01-6761363/086-2659833
FTAI

**KEARNEY, Ruth**
5 Beechlawn, South Hill Avenue,
Blackrock, Co Dublin.
Tel: 01-2833724
IFPP

**KEENAN, Marie**
Granada Institute,
Crinken House, Crinken Lane,
Shankill, Co Dublin.
Tel: 01-2721030
FTAI

**KEHOE, Helen**
11 Stockton Park,
Castleknock, Dublin 15.
Tel: 01-8216836
IAHIP

**KEIGHER, Marian**
Castle Street, Roscommon.
Tel: 0903-26124/26842
FTAI

**KELLEHER, Kathleen**
Mater Dei Counselling Centre,
Clonliffe Road, Dublin 3.
Tel: 01-8371892
FTAI

**KELLIHER, Anne**
8 Springfort, Montenotte, Cork
*and* 4 Cedar Court, Ashleigh Downs,
Tralee, Co Kerry.
Tel: 021-551031/066-7120142
IAHIP

**KELLY, Valerie**
21 Ballyboden Crescent,
Rathfarnham, Dublin 16
Tel: 01-4935803
FTAI

**KENNEDY, Jo**
Hesed House, 74 Tyrconnell Road,
Inchicore, Dublin 8.
Tel: 01-4549474
FTAI

**KENNY, Vincent**
c/o Vico, 2 Dungar Terrace,
Dun Laoghaire, Co Dublin
ICPA

**KIERNAN, Donal**
24 Parnell Road,
Bray, Co Wicklow.
Tel: 01-2868614/087-2319858
IAHIP

**KILCOYNE, Phyllis**
Ballaghaderreen, Co Roscommon.
Tel: 0907-61250
FTAI

**KILGALLEN, Aideen**
645 Riverforest,
Leixlip, Co Kildare
Tel: 01-6243514
IAHIP

**KILLORAN-GANNON, Sheila**
43 Belgrave Square,
Rathmines, Dublin 6.
Tel: 01-4960545
IAHIP

## KILMARTIN, Annie
The Healing House,
24 O'Connell Ave, Berkeley Road,
Dublin 7.
Tel: 01-2876141
IAHIP

## KIRK, Geraldine
Dept of Psychiatry,
Our Lady's Hospital,
Navan, Co Meath.
Tel: 046-72676
FTAI

## KLOPP, Marianne
15 Belmont Avenue,
Donnybrook, Dublin 4
Tel: 01-2692353
IAHIP

## KOHNSTAMM, Barbara
5 Tivoli Terrace East,
Dun Laoghaire, Co Dublin.
Tel: 01- 2803789
FTAI/IAHIP

## KRZECZUNOWICZ,
### Sarah E. (Kay)
2, Longwood Avenue,
off Sth. Circular Road, Dublin 8.
Tel: 01-4530344
IAHIP

## LALOR, Mary
Duile Counselling Psychotherapy
Centre, Maynooth Road,
Celbridge, Co Kildare.
Tel: 01-6273909
FTAI

## LANIGAN, NORA
c/o Arduna, 54 Clontarf Road,
Clontarf, Dublin 3.
Tel: 01-8332733 (W), 8318984
IAHIP

## LAWLOR, Mary Brigid
7 Hackett's Tce, St Luke's,
Cork.
Tel: 021-504339
IAHIP

## LEE, Mary
Vita House, Abbey Street,
Roscommon.
Tel: 0903-25898
FTAI

## LESLIE, Frank
7 Broadway Park,
Blanchardstown, Dublin 15.
Tel: 01-8214022
FTAI

## LEWIS, Maeve
New Day Counselling Centre,
11 Meath Street, Dublin 8.
Tel: 01-4547050
IAHIP

## LINDEN, Mairead
1 Ballinure Crescent,
Mahon, Cork.
Tel: 021-358372
IAHIP

## LINDSAY, John
Connect Associates,
Lonsdale House, Avoca Avenue,
Blackrock, Co Dublin.
Tel: 01-2884155
IAHIP

## LINDSAY, Susan
Connect Associates,
Lonsdale House, Avoca Avenue,
Blackrock, Co Dublin.
Tel: 01-2884155
IAHIP

LINNANE, Paul
Smithfield Chambers,
Smithfield, Dublin 7
Tel: 01-8173600
FTAI

LOGAN, Paddy
Percy Lane Psychotherapy,
56 Percy Lane,
Ballsbridge, Dublin 4.
Tel: 01-6675959
IAHIP

LONERGAN, Mary-Anna
108 Spring Road,
Letchworth, Herts SG6 3SL.
Tel: 01462-675694
IAHIP

LOUGHLIN, Paula
21 Cowper Road,
Rathmines, Dublin 6.
Tel: 01-4966766
IAHIP

LUCEY, Joe
Salesian Youth Enterprises,
72 Sean Mc Dermott Street, Dublin 1.
Tel: 01-8558792
ICPA

LYNCH, Barbara
Tus Nua, 43 Heather Lawn,
Marlay Wood,
Rathfarnham, Dublin 16
Tel: 01-4932244
IAHIP

LYNCH, Catherine
16 Ard na Meala,
Ballymun, Dublin 11.
Tel: 01-8426534
IAHIP

LYONS, Sheila
Stanhope Centre,
Lr Grangegorman Road, Dublin 7.
Tel: 01-6773965
FTAI

MAC GUINNESS, Irene
EHB, Basin Street,
Naas, Co Kildare.
Tel: 045-874066
FTAI

MAC NAMARA, Vincent
Eckhart House,
19 Clyde Road, Dublin 4.
Tel: 01-6684687
IAHIP

MAC NEILL, Sile
Baltyboys,
Blessington, Co Wicklow.
Tel: 045-867218
IAHIP

MADDEN, Joan
Knockanrawley Resource Centre,
Tipperary Town, Co Tipperary.
Tel: 062-52688
FTAI

MADDEN, Louise
Tigh na Feile, Ballygologue Rd,
Listowel, Co Kerry
Tel: 068-21156/086-8394981
IAHIP

MAGEE, David Louis
10 Park Villas,
Castleknock, Dublin 15.
Tel: 01-8211650
ICPA

MAGENIS, Maire
Regional Child & Family Health
Service, NWHB, General Hospital,
Letterkenny, Co Donegal.
Tel: 074-23563
FTAI

MAGUIRE, Maura
St John of God Hospital,
Stillorgan, Co Dublin and
Dunganstown, Wicklow, Co Wicklow
Tel: 086-2744474
FTAI

MAGUIRE, Una
Institute of Creative Counselling &
Psychotherapy,
82 Upper George's Street,
Dun Laoghaire, Co Dublin.
Tel: 01-2802523
IAHIP

MAHER, Ann
10 Forster Place,
Galway City.
Tel: 091-569129
IAHIP

MAHER, Bonnie
The Morehampton Clinic,
136 Morehampton Road,
Donnybrook, Dublin 4.
Tel: 01-4964799
IFPP

MAHER, Pascal
Greenlea Clinic, Greenlea Road,
Terenure, Dublin 6W.
Tel: 01-4502669
FTAI

MAIR, Bridget
37 Hermitage Grove,
Rathfarnham, Dublin 16
Tel: 01-4946942
IAHIP

MANDOS, Koos
Mater Child & Family Centre,
Ballymun Shopping Centre,
Dublin 11.
Tel: 01-8420319
FTAI

MANGAN, Mary
2 Harbour View, Summerhill North,
St Luke's, Cork
Tel: 021-505711
IAHIP

MANNION WALSHE,
  Deirdre
'Avalon', 8 Alma Park,
Monkstown Village, Co Dublin.
Tel: 01-2845208
IAHIP

MARTIN, Ray
Belgrave Avenue,
Wellington Road, Cork.
Tel: 021-505393
IAHIP

MASTERSON, Ingrid
'Alberta', Ardtona Avenue,
Lr. Churchtown Road, Dublin 14. and
76A Castlewood Gardens,
Pollerton Road, Carlow
Tel: 01-2988288
IFPP

MATHEWS, Peter
St Davnet's Hospital,
Monaghan, Co Monaghan.
Tel: 047-81822
CBT

MC ADAM, Frank
St Davnet's Hospital,
Monaghan, Co Monaghan.
Tel: 047-81822
CBT

## MC ALEER, Jennifer
Rosemount Centre,
60 Clare Street, Limerick.
Tel: 061-415697
FTAI

## MC CABE, Nancy
Dundalk Counselling Centre
Oakdene, 3 Seatown Place,
Dundalk, Co Louth
Tel: 042-9338333
IAHIP

## MC CARRICK, Tom
North Western Health Board,
Sligo.
Tel: 071-42111
IFPP

## MC CARTHY, Aine
15, Main Street,
Raheny, Dublin 5
Tel: 01-8318313
IAHIP

## MC CARTHY, Angela
Rape Crisis Centre,
70, Lr Leeson Street, Dublin 2
Tel: 01-6614911
IAHIP

## MC CARTHY, Anne
Limerick Social Service Centre,
Henry Street, Limerick.
Tel: 061-314111
IAHIP

## MC CARTHY, Imelda
Vico Consultation Centre,
2 Dungar Terrace,
Dun Laoghaire, Co Dublin.
Tel: 01-2843336
FTAI

## MC CARTHY, Rita
1 Newtown Villas, Newtown Avenue,
Blackrock, Co Dublin
Tel: 01-2832395
IFPP

## MC CARTHY, Ros
Clonsast,
Kilcock, Co Kildare.
Tel: 01-6287005
FTAI

## MC CONALOGUE, Margaret
Catherine Mc Auley Centre,
23 Herbert Street, Dublin 2
Tel: 01-6387500
FTAI

## MC CORMACK, Marijke
4 Pembroke Cottages, Pye Centre,
Dundrum, Dublin 16
Tel: 01-2962115
IAHIP

## MC COURT, Ann
Vico Consultation Centre,
Dungar Terrace,
Dun Laoghaire, Co Dublin
Tel: 01-2843336/01-2842992(H)
IAHIP

## MC COURT, Marie
206 Moyville,
Rathfarnham, Dublin 16.
Tel: 01-4945818
IAHIP

## MC DONNELL, Tricia
11 Bayside Square East,,
Sutton, Dublin 13.
Tel: 01-8395531
IAHIP

## MC FADDEN, Hugh
Tirconaill House, St Conal's Hospital,
Letterkenny, Co Donegal and
Sancta Maria, Gortlee,
Letterkenny, Co Donegal
Tel: 074-21919/074-23711
CBT

## MC GEE, Annette
Inst. of Psychosynthesis &
Transpersonal Theory,
Eckhart House,
19 Clyde Road, Dublin 4
Tel: 01-6684687
IAHIP

## MC GEE, Breda
35 Brompton Court, Dublin 15.
Tel: 01-8388077
FTAI

## MC GLYNN, Jim
North West Community Services,
Dungloe District Hospital,
Dungloe, Co Donegal.
Tel: 075-21044
CBT

## MC GOLDRICK, Mary
St Patrick's Hospital,
James' Street, Dublin 8.
Tel: 01-6775423
CBT

## MC GROARY-MEEHAN, Maureen
Donegal Community Services,
East End House,
Clar Road, Donegal Town.
Tel: 073-21933
CBT

## MC GUINNESS, Sharon
Markievcz House,
Sligo Mental Health Centre,
Barrack Street, Sligo
Tel: 071-55120
CBT

## MC HALE, Ed
66 Merrion Strand,
Sandymount, Dublin 4
Tel: 01-2698376
FTAI

## MC KEE, Anne
Lisgarode, Kilruane,
Nenagh, Co Tipperary and
2 Quin Street, Limerick
Tel: 067-32871
FTAI

## MC KEE, Maud
66 Manor Street, Dublin 7
Tel: 087-2424885
ICPA

## MC LEAVEY, Bernadette
12 Granville Crescent,
Cabinteely, Co Dublin.
Tel: 01-2847037
IAHIP

## MC LOUGHLIN, Maire
Kilrush Day Hospital, Co Clare
Tel: 065-9051559
FTAI

## MC LOUGHLIN, Sarah
Clanwilliam Institute,
18 Clanwilliam Terrace,
off Grand Canal Street, Dublin 2.
Tel: 01-6761363
FTAI

## MC MANUS, Libby
Rosemary Square,
Roscrea, Co Tipperary.
Tel: 0505-21222/21890
FTAI

## MC MORROW, Mary
Markievicz House,
Barrack Street, Sligo.
Tel: 071-55120
FTAI

## MEAGHER, Kathleen A.
Fortune House,
Cherry Orchard Hospital,
Dublin 10.
Tel: 087-2624140
IAHIP

## MEEK, Pauline
52 Dargle Road, Hollypark,
Blackrock, Co Dublin.
Tel: 01-2896435
FTAI

## MELVIN, Joan
108 Westbury,
Stillorgan, Co Dublin.
Tel: 01-2832940
IAHIP

## MERNAGH, Elizabeth
4 Pembroke Cottages, Pye Centre,
Ballinteer Road,
Dundrum, Dublin 16
Tel: 01-2966071
IAHIP

## MOHALLY, Derry
6 Sydney Place,
Wellington Road, Cork.
Tel: 021-507247
IAHIP

## MOLEY, Patrick
c/o Ladywell Centre,
Dundalk, Co Louth.
Tel: 042-9326156
FTAI

## MONAGHAN, Ann
Markievicz House, Sligo
Tel: 071-55120
FTAI

## MONAGHAN, Theresa
Aisling Centre,
37 Darling Street, Enniskillen,
Co Fermanagh.
Tel: 01365-325811
FTAI

## MOONEY MC GLOIN, Catherine
Cregg House,
Rosses Point Road, Sligo.
Tel: 071-77229
CBT

## MOORE, Lucy M.
Cluain Mhuire Family Centre,
Newtownpark Avenue,
Blackrock, Co Dublin.
Tel: 01-2833766
FTAI

## MOORE, Des
34 Lansdowne Park, Dublin 4
Tel: 01-6687386
CBT

## MORRISON, Anne
Markievicz House,
Barrack Street, Sligo.
Tel: 071-55120
FTAI

MORRISSEY, Germaine
10 Acorn Road,
Dundrum, Dublin 16
Tel: 01-2987364
IAHIP

MULHERE, Jacinta
St Vincent's Centre,
Navan Road, Dublin 7.
Tel: 01-8383234
CBT

MULHOLLAND,
  Marie Therese
St Patrick's Hospital,
James Street, Dublin 8.
Tel: 01-6775423
FTAI

MULLER, Elisabeth
Dalkey Avenue,
Dalkey, Co Dublin.
Tel: 01-2857185
IAHIP

MULLIGAN, Kathleen
Lissadell,
6 Hazelwood Grove, Dublin
Tel: 01-8472812
IAHIP

MURNANE, Eilis
12 Convent Lawns,
Ballyfermot, Dublin 10.
Tel: 01-6230898
FTAI

MURPHY, Ann C.
120 Leinster Road,
Dublin 6.
Tel: 01-4973080
IFPP

MURPHY, Brendan
Arduna,
54 Clontarf Road, Dublin 3.
Tel: 01-8332733/8331758
IFPP

MURPHY, David
119 Silchester Park,
Glenageary, Co Dublin.
Tel: 01-2303503
IAHIP

MURPHY, Ger
Institute of Creative Counselling &
Psychotherapy,
82 Upper George's Street,
Dun Laoghaire, Co Dublin.
Tel: 01-2802523
IAHIP

MURPHY, Mary
25 Glasnevin Hill,
Glasnevin, Dublin 9.
Tel: 01-8368966
FTAI

MURPHY, Mary
5, Ravenscourt, Donnybrook,
Douglas, Cork
Tel: 021-892377
IAHIP

MURPHY, Ruth
7, Albany Road, Ranelagh, Dublin 6
Tel: 01-4972969
FTAI

MURPHY, Trish
Clanwilliam Institute,
18, Clanwilliam Terrace,
Grand Canal Quay, Dublin 2
Tel: 01-6761363
FTAI

## MURPHY, Zoe
Arduna,
54, Clontarf Road, Dublin 3
Tel: 01-8332733
IFCAPP

## MURRAY, Denis
Fortune House,
Cherryorchard Hospital,
Cherryorchard, Dublin 10.
Tel: 01-6237356
FTAI

## MURRAY, Marie
St Vincent's Hospital,
Fairview, Dublin 3.
Tel: 01-8842430
FTAI

## MURRAY, Mary
24 Elmvale Court,
Wilton, Cork
Tel: 021-541854
IAHIP

## MYERS, Gerry
Ground Floor, 1 Church Street,
(Off John's Square), Limerick
*and*
1 St Flannan's St, Nenagh,
Co Tipperary.
Tel: 067-33280 / 086-8170380
IAHIP

## NANNERY, Teresa
The Lodge, Villa Nova,
Bundoran, Co Donegal *and*
General Hospital, Sligo
Tel: 072-41818/ 071-74644
IAHIP

## NAUGHTON, Annemarie
Lucena Clinic, Century Court,
100 Upper George's Street,
Dun Laoghaire, Co Dublin
Tel: 01-2809809
ICPA

## NEARY, Nora
Lucena Clinic, Century Court,
100 Upper George's Street,
Dun Laoghaire,,Co Dublin.
Tel: 01-2809809
IFCAPP

## NEWMAN, Josephine
Eckhart House,
19 Clyde Road, Dublin 4.
Tel: 01-6684687
IAHIP

## NÍ GHALLCHOBHAIR, Maighread
Benincasa,
1 Mount Merrion Avenue,
Blackrock, Co Dublin.
Tel: 01-2887066
IFCAPP

## NÍ NUALLÁIN, Máirín
Augustine Court,
Augustine Street, Galway.
Tel: 091-567035
IFPP

## NÍ UALLACHÁIN, Méabh
'St Louis', Blakestown Road,
Dublin 15.
Tel: 01-8217432
IAHIP

## NIC DHOMHNAILL, Caoimhe,
8 Alma Park, Monkstown Village, Co Dublin
Tel: 01-2303503
IFCAPP

## NOLAN, Bernadette
Seafield Lodge,
Stillorgan Road, Dublin 4.
Tel: 01-2693009
ICPA

## NOLAN, Inger
26 Longford Terrace,
Monkstown, Co Dublin.
Tel: 01-2809313
IAHIP/FTAI

## NOLAN, Patrick
26 Longford Terrace,
Monkstown, Co Dublin.
Tel: 01-2809313
IFPP/IAHIP

## NORMAND, Tessa
Various City Centre *and*
Dun Laoghaire, Co Dublin
Tel: 01-2801501
IAHIP

## NOWLAN, Kate
3, West End, Frome,
Somerset, BA11 3AD, England
Tel: 01373-471172 / 01373-464919
IFPP

## O'BRIEN, David.
Group Analytic Practice,
29 Lower Abbey Street, Dublin 1.
Tel: 01-8786486
IGAS

## O'BRIEN, Gay
93 Castleknock Park, Dublin 15.
Tel: 01-8217548
ICPA/FTAI

## O'BRIEN, Jim
St Brigid's Hospital,
Ardee, Co Louth.
Tel: 041-6853264
FTAI

## O'BRIEN, Margaret
6 Handpark, Rush, Co Dublin
FTAI

## O'BRIEN, Tom
Jonathan Swift Clinic, Dept of
Psychiatry, St James' Hospital,
Dublin 8.
Tel: 01-4537941 Ext. 2621
FTAI

## O'BRIEN, Valerie
Clanwilliam Institute,
18 Clanwilliam Terrace, Dublin 2.
Tel: 01-6762881
FTAI

## O'BYRNE, Celine
St Cynoc's Terrace, Ferbane,
Co Offaly, *and*
Tullamore Rape Crisis Centre,
10a, Patrick Street, Tullamore
Tel: 0902-54110
IAHIP

## O'CONNELL, Patricia
3 Farnhill Road,
Clonskeagh, Dublin 14
Tel: 01-2982994
IFCAPP

O'CONNOR, Aine
45 Huntstown Court,
Clonsilla, Dublin 15
Tel: 01-8216163
IAHIP

O'CONNOR, Colm J.
Cork & Ross Family Centre,
34 Paul Street, Cork.
Tel: 021-275678
FTAI

O'CONNOR, Karen E.
Fairview Therapy Centre,
10 Fairview Strand, Dublin 3.
Tel: 01-8561289
IAHIP

O'CONNOR, Marika
'Sanctuary', Lanesville,
Dun Laoghaire, Co Dublin.
Tel: 01-2809964
IAHIP

O'CONNOR, Mary Rose
Liberties College,
Bull Alley Street, Dublin 8
Tel: 01-4540044/82
IAHIP

O'DALAIGH, Liam
Claidhe Mor, Swords Road,
Santry, Dublin 9.
Tel: 01-8425955
FTAI

O'DEA, Catherine
Eglinton House,
Eglinton Terrace,
Dundrum, Dublin 14.
Tel: 01-2986204
IAHIP

O'DEA, Eileen
'Shalom' Therapy Suite,
5 Chapel Street,
Castlebar,Co Mayo.
Tel: 094-25142
FTAI

O'DOHERTY, Colm
ICCP,
82 Upper George's Street,
Dun Laoghaire, Co Dublin.
Tel: 01-2802523
IAHIP

O'DONNELL, Godfrey
Eastern Health Board,
140 St Laurence's Road,
Clontarf, Dublin 3.
Tel: 01-8338252
ICPA

O'DONNELL, Ruth
EHB, Strand House,
3 Philipsburgh Avenue,
Fairview, Dublin 3.
Tel: 01-8369899
FTAI

O'DONOGHUE, Eilis
3 Larkfield Gardens,
Harold's Cross, Dublin 6W
Tel: 01-4922653
IAHIP

O'DONOGHUE, Jim
Kedron, St Mary's Road,
Edenderry, Co Offaly *and*
Dublin Counselling & Therapy Centre,
41 Upr Gardiner Street, Dublin 1.
Tel: 0405-33311/01-8788236
IAHIP

## O'DONOGHUE, Paul
Dublin Counselling & Therapy
Centre,
41 Upr Gardiner Street, Dublin 1.
Tel: 01-8788236
IAHIP

## O'DONOVAN, Joan
Eckhart House,
19 Clyde Road, Dublin 4.
Tel: 01-6684687
IAHIP

## O'DONOVAN, Mairin
Cononagh House, Leap,
Skibbereen, Co Cork.
Tel: 028-33347
FTAI

## O'DONOVAN, Margot
5 Sycamore Walk,
Dublin 18.
Tel: 01-2849605
IAHIP

## O'DOWD, Maura
Cloonanorig House,
Cloonanorig,
Tralee, Co Kerry
Tel: 087-2618647
IAHIP

## O'DWYER, Mary
Mercy House,
Clonard Road, Wexford.
Tel: 053-23024
IAHIP

## O'FARRELL, Magda
Springfield Lodge, Ballybride Road,
Rathmichael, Co Dublin
Tel: 01-2822893
IAHIP

## O'FLAHERTY, Anne
St Louise's Unit,
Our Lady's Hospital,
Crumlin, Dublin 12.
Tel: 01-4558220
IFCAPP

## O'GRADY, Bernadette
Mercy Convent / Mercy College,
Woodford, Co Galway
Tel: 0509-49007/49076/49017
IAHIP

## O'GRADY, Ethna
Family Institute,
Ballaghaderreen, Co Roscommon.
Tel: 0907-61000
FTAI

## O'GRADY, Paul
Barnardos, Milbrook Lawns,
Dominic's Road, Tallaght, Dublin 24
Tel: 01-4627753
IFCAPP

## O'HANLON, Judy
Dundrum Gestalt Centre,
Park House, Eglington Terrace,
Upper Kilmacud Road, Dublin 14.
Tel: 01-2962015
IAHIP

## O'HARA, Carmel
Dublin 4 area.
Tel: 01-6601192
FTAI

## O'HORA, Claire
Greenlea Medical Centre,
Greenlea Road,
Terenure, Dublin 6.
Tel: 01-6680608
IFCAPP

**O'LEARY, Eleanor**
Dept. of Applied Psychology,
University College Cork.
Tel: 021-902612
IAHIP

**O'MAHONY, Berenice**
2 Herbert Park Lawn,
Gardiner's Hill, Cork
Tel: 021-502762
IAHIP

**O'MAHONY, Catherine**
Nationwide House,
Mullingar, Co Westmeath.
Tel: 044-61104
IFPP

**O'MAHONY, Eileen**
Cheeverstown House,
Templeogue, Dublin 12.
Tel: 01-4904681
FTAI

**O'MAHONY, Hank**
Baile Eamonn,
Spiddal, Co Galway
Tel: 091-553548
IAHIP

**O'MALLEY-DUNLOP, Ellen**
33 Springfield Road,
Terenure, Dublin 6W
Tel: 01-4904879
IFPP/IGAS/FTAI

**O'NEILL, Ann**
Fahy Law Offices,
John Street, Limerick.
Tel: 061-454736
IAHIP

**O'NEILL, Breege**
146 Seacrest,
Knocknacarra, Galway.
Tel: 091-591795
FTAI

**O'NEILL, Deborah**
Gurteenroe,
Bantry, Co Cork
Tel: 027-52193
IAHIP

**O'NEILL, Elizabeth**
Mid Western Health Board,
ACC House, Pearse Street,
Nenagh, Co Tipperary.
Tel: 067-31212
FTAI

**O'NEILL, Julia**
Aughinish,
Kinvarra, Co Galway.
Tel: 065-7078252
IAHIP

**O'NEILL, Mary**
New Day Counselling Centre,
11 Meath Street, Dublin 8.
Tel: 01-4547050
IAHIP

**O'NEILL, Nora**
7 Woodbrook,
Rochestown Road, Cork.
Tel: 021-362068
IAHIP

**O'REILLY, Joseph**
Ferryhouse,
Clonmel, Co Tipperary.
Tel: 052-24633
IAHIP

## O'ROURKE, Darina
4 Pembroke Cottages,
Pye Centre, Ballinteer Road,
Dundrum, Dublin 14.
Tel: 01-4902514
IAHIP

## O'SCOLLAIN, Eibhlin
St John of God Hospital,
Stillorgan, Co Dublin.
Tel: 01-2881781 Ext. 252
FTAI

## O'SHAUGHNESSY, Marie
Hesed House, 74 Tyrconnell Road,
Inchicore, Dublin 8.
Tel: 01-4549474
FTAI

## O'SHEA, Deirdre
St Clare's Unit, The Children's
Hospital,
Temple Street, Dublin 1
Tel: 01-8745214
FTAI

## O'SULLIVAN, Ann
18 Upper Mallow Street, Limerick
Tel: 061-327717
IAHIP

## O'SULLIVAN, Bernadette
Vico Consultation Centre,
2 Dungar Terrace,
Dun Laoghaire, Co Dublin
Tel: 01-2843336
ICPA / FTAI

## O'SULLIVAN, Creina
Mary Street Medical Centre,
Mary Street,
Dungarvan, Co Waterford.
Tel: 058-45911
FTAI

## O'SULLIVAN, Marych
33 Woodquay, Galway.
Tel: 091-567511
IFPP/IFCAPP

## O'SULLIVAN, Rita
Rutland Centre,
Knocklyon, Dublin 16.
Tel: 01-4946358
IAHIP

## O'TOOLE, Muriel
6 Pepper's Court,
Portlaoise, Co Laois.
Tel: 0502-62101
IAHIP

## OWENS, Conor
Lucena Clinic, Blessington Road,
Tallaght, Dublin 24.
Tel: 01-4526333
IFCAPP

## PARKS, Ann
Dundalk Counselling Centre,
'Oakdene', 3 Seatown Place,
Dundalk, Co Louth.
Tel: 042-9338333
IAHIP

## PEAKIN, Anne
1 Woodlawn, Upr Churchtown Road,
Dundrum, Dublin 14.
Tel: 01-2959043
IAHIP

## PERREM, Breda
3 Sydenham Terrace,
Monkstown, Co Cork
Tel: 021-842087
IAHIP

DIRECTORY

**PHALAN, Sally**
1 Athgoe Drive,
Shankill, Co Dublin *and*
Waterfall Road,
Enniskerry, Co Wicklow
Tel: 01-2829251
IFCAPP

**PORTER, Sheila**
5 Westerton Rise,
Dundrum, Dublin 16.
Tel: 01-2987870
FTAI

**PRENDERVILLE, Mary**
9 Albany Road,
Ranelagh, Dublin 6.
Tel: 01-4973425
IAHIP

**PRICE, Noeleen M.**
Higginstown,
Slane, Co Meath
Tel: 041-9824576
FTAI

**PRYLE, Fiona**
Catherine McAuley Centre,
23 Herbert Street, Dublin 2.
Tel: 01-6387546
FTAI

**PYLE, Mary**
31 Palmerstown Road, Dublin 6.
Tel: 01-4973670
IFPP

**RICHARDSON, Anne**
St Patrick's Hospital,
James' Street, Dublin 8.
Tel: 01-6775423
FTAI

**RICHARDSON, Colette**
5/36 Boundary Road,
London NW8 OHG,
Tel: 0171-372 4886
FTAI

**RIGNEY, Jeanette**
Tabor Counselling & Therapy Centre,
316 The Lawns, Belgard Heights,
Tallaght, Dublin 24
Tel: 01-4518869
IAHIP

**RINTOUL, Irene**
Inst. of Creative Counselling &
Psychotherapy,
82 Upr George's Street,
Dun Laoghaire, Co Dublin
Tel: 01-2802523
IAHIP

**RIORDAN, Gillian**
Eckhart House,
19 Clyde Road, Dublin 4.
Tel: 01-6684687
IAHIP

**ROCHE, Anne**
Oasis Counselling, St Laurence's Place E.,
Seville Place, Dublin 1
Tel: 01-8364524
IAHIP

**ROCHE, Declan**
Clanwilliam Institute,
18 Clanwilliam Terrace,
Grand Canal Quay, Dublin 2.
Tel: 01- 6762881
FTAI

**ROCHE, Freda**
46, Elmwood Avenue Lr,
Ranelagh, Dublin 6
Tel: 01-4971188 / 4971722
FTAI

ROCHE, Sile
Stanhope Centre,
Lr Grangegorman, Dublin 7.
Tel: 01-6773965
FTAI

ROE, Liam
3 Rowan Close, Castletown,
Celbridge, Co Kildare.
Tel: 01- 6271301
FTAI

ROTHERY, Nuala
Psychology Department,
Trinity College, Dublin 2.
Tel: 01-6081489
IAHIP

RUSSELL, Maura
Rutland Centre,
Knocklyon House,
Knocklyon Road, Dublin 16.
Tel: 01-4946358
ICPA

RUTH-MURRAY, Ann M.
Shoni, Well Road,
Little Island, Cork and
35 Woodquay, Galway
Tel: 021-354843
IAHIP

RYAN, Anne
Dublin Counselling & Therapy
Centre,
41 Upr Gardiner Street, Dublin 1.
Tel: 01-8788236
IAHIP

RYAN, Anne
6 Beech Park, Blackrock,
Dundalk, Co Louth
Tel: 042-9322590
IAHIP

RYAN, Catherine
4 Pembroke Cottages, Pye Centre,
Ballinteer Road,
Dundrum, Dublin 14.
Tel: 01-2962115
IAHIP

RYAN, David.
St Helen's, York Road,
Dun Laoghaire, Co Dublin
Tel: 01-2801214(W)/2845317(H)
IAHIP

RYAN, Derval
Aer Lingus Employee Assistance,
Personnel Building,
Dublin Airport, Co Dublin.
Tel: 01-8862868
IFPP/IGAS

RYAN, Mairead
Clifton House,
Lr Fitzwilliam Street, Dublin 2.
Tel: 01-6614828
CBT

RYAN, Teresa
Warrenmount Centre,
Blackpitts, Dublin 8.
Tel: 01-4542622
IAHIP

RYAN, Toni
An Cosan, Jobstown,
Tallaght, Dublin 24.
Tel: 01-4582194(W)/4922447(H)
IAHIP

SAHAFI, Janet E.
Naas, Co Kildare.
Tel: 045-894187
IAHIP

## SAMPSON, Annie
Kilcornan,
Kilkishen, Co Clare
Tel: 061-367035 / 086-2320525
IAHIP

## SCIASCIA, Dolores
34 Shoreside, Cullinagh,
Ballina/Killaloe, Co Tipperary
Tel: 061-375171
FTAI

## SCULLY, Mary
Connolly Norman House,
224 North Circular Road, Dublin 7
Tel: 01-8681400
FTAI

## SCULLY, Patricia
Stanhope Centre, (EHB),
Grangegorman Lower, Dublin 7.
Tel: 01-6773965/087-2385027
FTAI

## SCULLY, Ros
No 1 Wine Street, Sligo
Tel: 071-77702
IAHIP

## SELL, Patrick
Centre for Biodynamic & Integrative
Psychotherapy, Tracht Beach,
Kinvara, Co Galway.
Tel: 091-637192
IAHIP

## SHEEHAN, Jim
6 Windsor Road, Dublin 6.
Tel: 01-4964406
FTAI

## SHEEHAN, Mary
St Brendan's Hospital,
3 Orchard View,
Rathdown Road, Dublin 7.
Tel: 01-8383851
IFPP

## SHEEHAN, Tom
Psychology Department
Roscommon Community Care,
Ardsallagh,
Athlone Road, Roscommon.
Tel: 0903-27089
FTAI

## SHEILL, Mary
Solace,
36 Dublin Street, Carlow.
Tel: 0503-30611
IAHIP

## SHERIDAN, Anne
'Greenlands',
Golf Course Road,
Letterkenny, Co Donegal.
Tel: 074-27707
FTAI

## SHIELDS, Vivienne
46 Elmwood Avenue,
Ranelagh, Dublin 6.
Tel: 01-4971188/4971722
FTAI

## SHORTEN, Karen Ilean
28 Parkwood Grove,
Aylesbury, Dublin 24.
Tel: 01-4514637
IAHIP

## SKAR, Patricia
12 Brook Court,
Monkstown, Co. Dublin.
Tel: 01-2300577
IFPP

SKELTON, Ross
14 Gledswood Avenue,
Clonskeagh, Dublin 14.
Tel: 01-2697682
IFPP

SMITH, Ray
Group Analytic Practice,
Global House,
29 Lr Abbey Street, Dublin 1.
Tel: 01-8786486
IGAS

SMITH, Susan
25 Glasnevin Hill, Dublin 9.
Tel: 01-8368966
FTAI

SMYTH, Geraldine
Eckhart House,
19 Clyde Road, Dublin 4.
Tel: 01-4923430 (H) / 6684687 (W)
IAHIP

SOMERS, Olive
Group Analytic Practice,
Global House,
29 Lr Abbey Street, Dublin 1.
Tel: 01-8786486
IGAS

SPARROW, Bobbie
Galway City Centre, Galway.
Tel: 091-589464
IAHIP

STONE, William
1 Church Street, IFAC House, (Off
John's Square,, Limerick.
Tel: 061-315478
IAHIP

SWAIN, Ronny
Dept of Applied Psychology,
University College, Cork
Tel: 021-902503
IAHIP

SWEENEY, Brion
2nd Floor, Phibsboro Tower,
Phibsboro, Dublin 7.
Tel: 01- 8820300
ICPA

SWEENEY, Delma
1 Olney Mews,
Rathgar Avenue, Dublin 6.
Tel: 01-4966657
IAHIP

SWEENEY, Irene M.
Vico Consultation Centre,
2 Dungar Terrace,
Dun Laoghaire, Co Dublin
Tel: 01:2843336
IFPP

SWEENEY, Patrick
Presbytery 2,
Dunmanus Road,
Cabra West, Dublin 7.
Tel: 01-8389525
FTAI

TIERNEY, Maggie
'Kilmoremoy', Friarstown,
Ballyclough, Co Limerick.
Tel: 061-229143
IAHIP

TONE, Yvonne
St Patrick's Hospital,
James' Street, Dublin 8.
Tel: 01-6775423
CBT

**TROOP, Deborah**
31 Castle Park,
Monkstown, Co Dublin.
Tel: 01-2806321
IAHIP/FTAI

**TYRRELL, Patricia M.**
New Government Buildings,
Anne Street, Wexford.
Tel: 053-24812(W)/38349(H)
FTAI

**UNDERWOOD-QUINN,**
  **Nicola**
19 Sandymount Road, Dublin 4.
Tel: 01-6684611
FTAI/IAHIP

**VAN DOORSLAER, Mia**
Vico Consultation Centre,
2 Dungar Terrace,
Northumberland Avenue,
Dun Laoghaire, Co Dublin.
Tel: 01-2843336
ICPA

**VAN HOUT, Els**
Skodsborgvej 189, 2850 Naerum,
Copenhagen, Denmark.
Tel: 00-45-45.80.83.55
IAHIP

**WADE, Richard A.**
11 The Rise, Mount Merrion,
Blackrock, Co Dublin
Tel: 01-2881012
ICPA

**WALL MURPHY, Maura**
2 Shanganagh Vale,
Cabinteely, Dublin 18.
Tel: 01-2824024
FTAI

**WALLACE, Carmel**
93 Elm Mount Park,
Beaumont, Dublin 9.
Tel: 01-8463136/8317782
IAHIP

**WALLACE, George**
5 Castle Close,
Mahon, Cork.
Tel: 021-358206
IAHIP

**WALSH, Angela**
324 Richmond Court,
Richmond Avenue South,
Dartry, Dublin 6.
Tel: 01-4961039
FTAI

**WALSH, Mary-Paula**
Turning Point, 23 Crofton Road,
Dun Laoghaire, Co Dublin.
Tel: 01-2800626/2807888
IAHIP/ICPA

**WALSH, Tony**
Inst of Psychosocial Medicine,
2 Eden Park, Summerhill Road,
Dun Laoghaire, Co Dublin
Tel: 01-2800084
ICPA

**WARD, Mary**
Woodquay, Galway.
Tel: 091-844148
IAHIP

**WARD, Shirley A.**
'Amethyst', 28 Beech Court,
Killiney, Co Dublin.
Tel: 01-2850976
IAHIP

WARDEN, Norman
Cnocan An Bhodaigh,
Furbo, Co Galway.
Tel: 091-591443
IAHIP

WATSON, Patricia
Barra, Balkill Road,,
Howth, Co Dublin
Tel: 01-8322472
IAHIP

WEATHERILL, Rob
12 Crosthwaite Park East,
Dun Laoghaire, Co Dublin
Tel: 01-2805332
IFPP

WHITE, Joan
2 Dungar Terrace,
Dun Laoghaire, Co Dublin.
Tel: 01-2843336(W)/2844044(H)
FTAI

WHYTE, Monica
Alcohol Treatment Unit,
Baggot St Community Hospital,
18 Upr Baggot Street, Dublin 4.
Tel: 01-6607838
FTAI

WIECZOREK-DEERING,
   Dorit
School of Social Sciences,
DIT, Rathmines House, Dublin 6.
Tel: 01-4023509
IFCAPP

WILLIAMS, Jane
Vico Consultation Centre, 2 Dungar
Terrace,
Dun Laoghaire, Co Dublin
Tel: 01-2843336
FTAI

WILSDON, Sheelagh
c/o 26 Longford Terrace,
Monkstown, Co Dublin
Tel: 087-6967389
IFPP

WOODS, Jean
Dundalk Counselling Centre,
'Oakdene', 3 Seatown Place,
Dundalk, Co Louth.
Tel: 042-9338333
IAHIP

WRIXON GOGGIN, Pauline
Aherina,
Kilmore, Co Clare.
Tel: 061-473269
IAHIP

YOUNG, Anne
27 Rostrevor Road,
Rathgar, Dublin 6
Tel: 01-4970331
IFPP

YOUNG, Sheilagh M.
2 The Coppins,
Foxrock, Dublin 18.
Tel: 01-2892287
FTAI.

# PART IV

# A Directory by County
# of Psychotherapists in Ireland

*For addresses and telephone numbers, please refer to the Directory section*

## ANTRIM
BURNS, Maura
HORNER, Carol

## ARMAGH
HORNER, Philomena

## CARLOW
FADDEN, Rosaleen
MASTERSON, Ingrid
SHEILL, Mary

## CAVAN
BROWNE, Essie

## CLARE
COLLINS, Geraldine
HUNTER, Alison I.
MC LOUGHLIN, Maire
SAMPSON, Annie
WRIXON GOGGIN,
   Pauline

## CORK
AYLWIN, Susan
BRIGHT, Jill
BROWNE, Larry
CONNOLLY, Brendan M.

CUNNINGHAM, Kathy
DEVLIN, Fiona
DOYLE, Mary
ELLIS, Mary
FINLAYSON, Douglas
FLYNN, Stephen
FRYER, Anthony
GROVER, Mary
HARRINGTON, Eileen
HEGARTY, Tony
HERLIHY, Marie
HOLLAND, Joanna
JACKSON, Ann
JONES, Coleen
KELLIHER, Anne
LAWLOR, Mary Brigid
LINDEN, Mairead
MANGAN, Mary
MARTIN, Ray
MOHALLY, Derry
MURPHY, Mary
MURRAY, Mary
O'CONNOR, Colm J.
O'DONOVAN, Mairin
O'LEARY, Eleanor
O'MAHONY, Berenice
O'NEILL, Deborah

O'NEILL, Nora
PERREM, Breda
RUTH-MURRAY, Ann M.
SWAIN, Ronny
WALLACE, George

## DONEGAL

DEENY, Peggy
DEVLIN, Teresa
FINNEGAN, Leo
MAGENIS, Maire
MC FADDEN, Hugh
MC GLYNN, Jim
MC GROARY-MEEHAN,
   Maureen
NANNERY, Teresa
SHERIDAN, Anne

## DOWN

BENSON, Jarlath F.

## DUBLIN

ANDREWS, Paul
ARNOLD, Mavis
ARTHURS, Mary
BAILEY, Jane
BAIRD, Jane
BAYLY, Kathrin
BERMINGHAM, Anne
   Marie
BERMINGHAM, Paula
BEAUMONT, Margaret
BOLAND, Emille
BOYLE, Martin
BOYNE, Edward
BREEN, Noreen

BREEN, Thomas
BROPHY, John
BROPHY, Margaret T.M.
BURKE, Phil
BURSTALL, Taru
BUTLER, Goretti
BUTLER, Maggie
BYRNE, Carmel
BYRNE, Nollaig
CADWELL, Nuala
CALLANAN, Fiodhna
CALLANAN, William
CAMPBELL, Carmel
CANAVAN, Mary
CARBERRY, Brian
CARR, Alan
CARROLL, Anna
CARROLL, Patricia
CARTON, Simone
CASEY, Grainne
CASSERLY, Felicity
CHILDERS, Nessa
CLAFFEY, Elaine
CLARKE, Margaret
CLARKE, Michele
COGHLAN, Helena
COLEMAN, Padraig
COLGAN, Patrick J.
COLLEARY, Maura
COLLINS, Barbara
COLLINS, Deirdre
COLLINS, Ines
CONAGHAN, Mary
CONNOLLY, Margaret,
CONROY, Kay
COX, Ann

COX CAMERON, Olga
COYLE, Brigid
CULLEN, Mary
DALY, Margaret
DALY, Martin
DALY, Martin J.
DAVEY, Damien
DE BURCA, Bairbre
DE JONGH, Corry
DE LACY, Mara
DELMONTE, Michael M.
DENNEHY, Noreen
DIBBLE, Annie
DILLON, Marie T.
DOCKERY, Bernadette
DONNELLY, Patricia
DONOGHUE, Mary
DOOLEY, Deirdre
DOWD, Teresa
DOYLE, Rosaleen
DOYLE, Sherry
DRISCOLL, Angela
DUFFY, Mary
DUGGAN, Colman
DUNLEA, Marian
DWYER, Frankie-Ann
EGAN, Angela
FAHY, Bernadette
FAY, Joe
FITZGERALD, Barbara
FLEMING, Pearl
FLYNN, Deirdre
FLYNN, Madeleine
FOLEY, Dermot
FOLEY, Robert
FORBES, Jean

FORREST, Mary
FOX, Michael
FOY, Emma
FULTON, Linda
GAFFNEY, Delia
GALLIGAN, Claire
GALLIGAN, Patricia
GARLAND, Clive
GILL, Anne
GILLILAND, Kay P.
GILMARTIN, Helen
GLEESON, Betty
GORDON, Evelyn
GRIMLEY, Carmel
GRINDLEY, Geraldine M.
GROSSMAN FREYNE, Gail
GUNNE, Dorothy
HARGIN, Mary Rose
HARNEY, Vivian
HAUGHEY, Monica
HAYES, Fran
HEFFERNAN, Michael
HEGARTY, Donal
HEGARTY, Owen
HENNIGAN, Cecily
HOLLAND, Mary
HONNAY, Emiel
HOULIHAN, Tom
HOWLETT, Brian
JACKSON, Caitriona
JEBB, Winston
JEFFRIES, Mary
JENNINGS, Norman
JONES, Helen
JOYCE, Nora
JUDGE, Jimmy

JUTHAN, Kay
KEANE, Verena
KEARNEY, Philip
KEARNEY, Ruth
KEENAN, Marie
KEHOE, Helen
KELLEHER, Kathleen
KELLY, Valerie
KENNEDY, Jo
KENNY, Vincent
KILLORAN-GANNON,
  Sheila
KILMARTIN, Annie
KLOPP, Marianne
KOHNSTAMM, Barbara
KRZECZUNOWICZ, Sarah
  E. (Kay)
LANIGAN, Nora
LESLIE, Frank
LEWIS, Maeve
LINDSAY, John
LINDSAY, Susan
LINNANE, Paul
LOGAN, Paddy
LOUGHLIN, Paula
LUCEY, Joe
LYNCH, Barbara
LYNCH, Catherine
LYONS, Sheila
MACNAMARA, Vincent
MAGEE, David Louis
MAGUIRE, Maura
MAGUIRE, Una
MAHER, Bonnie
MAHER, Pascal
MAIR, Bridget

MANDOS, Koos
MANNION WALSHE,
  Deirdre
MASTERSON, Ingrid
MC CARTHY, Aine
MC CARTHY, Angela
MC CARTHY, Imelda
MC CARTHY, Rita
MC CONALOGUE,
  Margaret
MC CORMACK, Marijke
MC COURT, Ann
MC COURT, Marie
MC DONNELL, Tricia
MC GEE, Annette
MC GEE, Breda
MC GOLDRICK, Mary
MC HALE, Edmund
MC KEE, Maud
MC LEAVEY, Bernadette
MC LOUGHLIN, Sarah
MEAGHER, Kathleen A.
MEEK, Pauline
MELVIN, Joan
MERNAGH, Elizabeth.
MOORE, Des
MOORE, Lucy M
MORRISSEY, Germaine.
MULHERE, Jacinta
MULHOLLAND, Marie
  Therese
MULLER, Elisabeth
MULLIGAN, Kathleen
MURNANE, Eilis
MURPHY, Ann.
MURPHY, Brendan

MURPHY, David
MURPHY, Ger
MURPHY, Mary
MURPHY, Ruth
MURPHY, Trish
MURPHY, Zoe
MURRAY, Denis
MURRAY, Marie
NAUGHTON, Annemarie
NEARY, Nora
NEWMAN, Josephine
NÍ GHALLCHOBHAIR,
  Maighréad
NÍ UALLACHÁIN, Méabh
NIC DHOMHNAILL,
  Caoimhe
NOLAN, Bernadette
NOLAN, Inger
NOLAN, Patrick
NORMAND, Tessa
O'BRIEN, David
O'BRIEN, Gay
O'BRIEN, Margaret
O'BRIEN, Tom
O'BRIEN, Valerie
O'CONNELL, Patricia
O'CONNOR, Aine
O'CONNOR, Karen E.
O'CONNOR, Marika
O'CONNOR, Mary Rose
O'DALAIGH, Liam
O'DEA, Catherine
O'DOHERTY, Colm
O'DONNELL, Godfrey
O'DONNELL, Ruth
O'DONOGHUE, Eilis

O'DONOGHUE, Jim
O'DONOGHUE, Paul
O'DONOVAN, Joan
O'DONOVAN, Margot
O'FARRELL, Magda
O'FLAHERTY, Anne
O'GRADY, Paul
O'HANLON, Judy
O'HARA, Carmel
O'HORA, Claire
O'MAHONY, Eileen
O'MALLEY-DUNLOP, Ellen
O'NEILL, Mary
O'ROURKE, Darina
O'SCOLLAIN, Eibhlin
O'SHAUGHNESSY, Marie
O'SHEA, Deirdre
O'SULLIVAN, Bernadette
O'SULLIVAN, Rita
OWENS, Conor
PEAKIN, Anne
PHALAN, Sally
PORTER, Sheila
PRENDERVILLE, Mary
PRYLE, Fiona M.
PYLE, Mary
RICHARDSON, Anne
RIGNEY, Jeanette
RINTOUL, Irene
RIORDAN, Gillian
ROCHE, Anne
ROCHE, Declan
ROCHE, Freda
ROCHE, Sile
ROTHERY, Nuala
RUSSELL, Maura

RYAN, Anne
RYAN, Catherine
RYAN, David
RYAN, Derval
RYAN, Mairead
RYAN, Teresa
RYAN, Toni
SCULLY, Mary
SCULLY, Patricia
SHEEHAN, Jim
SHEEHAN, Mary
SHIELDS, Vivienne
SHORTEN, Karen Ilean
SKAR, Patricia
SKELTON, Ross
SMITH, Ray
SMITH, Susan
SMYTH, Geraldine
SOMERS, Olive
SWEENEY, Brion
SWEENEY, Delma
SWEENEY, Irene M.
SWEENEY, Patrick
TONE, Yvonne
TROOP, Deborah
UNDERWOOD-QUINN,
   Nicola
VAN DOORSLAER, Mia
WADE, Richard A.
WALL MURPHY, Maura
WALLACE, Carmel
WALSH, Angela
WALSH, Mary-Paula
WALSH, Tony
WARD, Shirley A.
WATSON, Patricia

WEATHERILL, Rob
WHITE, Joan
WHYTE, Monica
WIECZOREK-DEERING,
   Dorit
WILLIAMS, Jane
WILSDON, Sheelagh
YOUNG, Anne
YOUNG, Sheilagh

## FERMANAGH
MONAGHAN, Theresa

## GALWAY
BREHONY, Rita
BROSNAN, Joan
BUCKLEY, Marguerite
CONNEELY, Caitlin
DELAHUNTY, Alan
DENENY, Mary
DRISCOLL, Zelie
DUGGAN, Noël
FAHY, Michael
FRAWLEY, Angela
FRAWLEY, Michael
GRIEVE, Karin
HESKIN, Christina
JACKSON, Caitriona
MAHER, Ann
NÍ NUALLÁIN, Máirín
O'GRADY, Bernadette
O'MAHONY, Hank
O'NEILL, Breege
O'NEILL, Julia
O'SULLIVAN, Marych
RUTH-MURRAY, Ann

SELL, Patrick
SPARROW, Bobbie
WARD, Mary B.
WARDEN, Norman

### KERRY

BYRNE, Patrick
FITZGERALD, Ann
KELLIHER, Anne
MADDEN, Louise
O'DOWD, Maura

### KILDARE

BOGGINS, Tom
BUCKLEY, Marion
CAHILL, Michele
CONNOLLY, Brendan
FITZMAURICE, John
HARGIN, Mary Rose
KILGALLEN, Aideen
LALOR, Mary
MAC GUINNESS, Irene
MC CARTHY, Ros
ROE, Liam
SAHAFI, Janet E.

### KILKENNY

FINGLETON, May

### LAOIS

BANNON, John
BERGIN, Alexander
FINGLETON, May
O'TOOLE, Muriel

### LIMERICK

COLLINS-SMYTH,
  Margaret
CUNNINGHAM, Nora
DOYLE, Grainne
MC ALEER, Jennifer
MC CARTHY, Anne
MC KEE, Anne
MYERS, Gerry
O'NEILL, Ann
O'SULLIVAN, Ann
STONE, William
TIERNEY, Maggie

### LONGFORD

BEIRNE, Rosarii

### LOUTH

COSTELLO, Margaret
DEERY, Patrick
DULLAGHAN, Elizabeth
  (Lillie)
DUNNE, Patricia
HOWARD, Leslie
MC CABE, Nancy
MOLEY, Patrick
O'BRIEN, Jim
PARKS, Ann
RYAN, Anne
WOODS, Jean B.

### MAYO

BRENT, Rebecca
DUFFY, Kathleen
FORDE, Angela
FRENCH, Gerry
O'DEA, Eileen

## MEATH
DUFFY, Martin
FOLEY, Miriam A.
FRENCH, Gerry
HONNAY, Emiel
KIRK, Geraldine
PRICE, Noeleen M.

## MONAGHAN
BURBRIDGE, Paul
MATHEWS, Peter
MC ADAM, Frank

## OFFALY
O'BYRNE, Celine
O'DONOGHUE, Jim

## ROSCOMMON
KEIGHER, Marian
KILCOYNE, Phyllis
LEE, Mary
O'GRADY, Ethna
SHEEHAN, Tom

## SLIGO
BARRY, Kathleen
CURTIN, Gerardine
DOHERTY, Myra
GUNNE, David
HIRST, Iain
MC CARRICK, Tom
MC GUINNESS, Sharon
MC MORROW, Mary
MONAGHAN, Ann
MOONEY MC GLOIN,
   Catherine

MORRISON, Anne
NANNERY, Teresa
SCULLY, Ros

## TIPPERARY
BOURKE, Carmel
DOWNEY, Betty
DUNCAN, Audrey
MADDEN, Joan
MC KEE, Anne
MC MANUS, Libby
MYERS, Gerry
O'NEILL, Elizabeth
O'REILLY, Joseph
SCIASCIA, Dolores

## TYRONE
DEENY, Peggy

## WATERFORD
BYRNE, Ruth
FRASER, Teresa
O'SULLIVAN, Creina

## WESTMEATH
BENNETT, Eamonn
O'MAHONY, Catherine

## WEXFORD
HILL, Rosemary
O'DWYER, Mary
TYRRELL, Patricia M.

## WICKLOW
CARROLL, Patricia
COLLINS, Mary

COUNTY DIRECTORY

DUNNE, Ann Maria
EGAN, Barbara
KIERNAN, Donal
MAC NEILL, Sile
MAGUIRE, Maura
PHALAN, Sally

### ENGLAND
LONERGAN, Mary-Anna

NOWLAN, Kate
RICHARDSON, Colette

### DENMARK
VAN HOUT, Els

### ISLE OF MAN
BYRNE, Tim